FIRESIDE

VITAMINS IN YOUR LIFE

And the Micronutrients
(Trace Elements)

YOU CAN'T LIVE WITHOUT THEM!

by Erwin Di Cyan, Ph.D.

With a Preface by
Chauncey D. Leake, Ph.D., Sc.D.

A Fireside Book
Published by Simon and Schuster

A Fireside Book
Published by Simon and Schuster
A Division of Gulf & Western Corporation
Simon & Schuster Building
Rockefeller Center, 1230 Avenue of the Americas
New York, New York 10020
FIRESIDE and colophon are
trademarks of Simon & Schuster

ISBN 0-671-21711-9
ISBN 0-671-22010-1 Pbk.
Library of Congress Catalog Card Number 73–21473
Designed by Irving Perkins
Manufactured in the United States of America

5   6   7   8   9   10   11

8   9   10   11   Pbk.

ACKNOWLEDGMENTS

To Peter Schwed, chairman of the board of editors of Simon and Schuster, my publisher, I am grateful for sound suggestions which improved the book by making vital information more accessible and for his encouragement. To Mrs. Margaret Markham and Miss Arline Harris I owe thanks for their help in supplying me with many useful items from the literature. I am also thankful to Mrs. Michele A. Friedman for her patience in the expert typing of the manuscript despite the frequent and complex changes I made during the process. Also, I acknowledge the courtesy of Pyramid Publications, Inc., for permission to use portions from one of my previous books, *Vitamin E and Aging*. And I want to express my appreciation to both Professor Philip H. Miele and Jean-Louis Brindamour, Ph.D., for their encouragement, and to Mrs. Margaret F. O'Connell for editorial advice.

E.D.

DEDICATED with love
to my son, Adrian Burke Di Cyan;
my daughter, Erika Di Cyan Hessman,
and her husband, Lawrence Hessman, M.D.;
and in memory of my wife,
Lucille Di Cyan.

November 1973

Good nutrition is a matter of adequate selection among the various nutrients that foods supply. It is *not* a fixation on vitamins, minerals, micronutrients, lecithin, nor on any specific vegetable, fruit, or any other single foodstuff.

Think first in terms of *food*, supplementing your diet judiciously with vitamins and micronutrients—not the other way around.

CONTENTS

FOREWORD

FOR INTELLIGENT PEOPLE generally, this clear and brief account of vitamins and micronutrients (or trace minerals) should be very welcome. It provides a concise summary of the significant information now available. It should be a useful guide.

Most people in cultured countries know something about vitamins, or think they do, but they are not likely to be appropriately informed on micronutrients. Even to those who think they know about vitamins and micronutrients, it may come as something of a surprise to discover that there are so many vitamins (13 that are well established) and so many micronutrients (some 15 are now recognized).

Actually there may be more micronutrients of whose significance we are not yet certain. It is even possible that in all the long process of evolution, all of the 103 or so recognized elements have found some role in living activity.

Some elements such as sodium, potassium, and calcium, as well as chlorine, phosphorus, and sulfur, are used by living things in relatively large amounts. Carbon is an element present in all organic material and in great abundance in plants and animals.

Humans utilize large amounts of nitrogen in foods, and we require oxygen continually. Furthermore we are all subjected, in civilized communities, to possible poisoning with such elements as arsenic, cadmium, chromium, mercury, lead, bismuth, beryllium, or barium. Even lithium, boron, and aluminum may readily enough get into our bodies and produce some effect or other. It would seem, thus, that in our evolutionary development we

11

have tended to have contact with all the chemical elements in our environment.

Our nutritional knowledge of vitamins and micronutrients is relatively recent. Sir Frederick Gowland Hopkins (1861–1947) first gave clear evidence of the importance of "accessory factors" in normal dietaries in 1912. About the same time, Casimir Funk (1884–1969) first used the word *vitamine*. He thought that these accessory factors were chemical amines. The word was later changed to *vitamin,* since many of these accessory factors were found to be chemically distinct from amines.

The fat-soluble vitamin A was discovered in 1913 by Elmer Verner McCollum (1879–1971). The separation of vitamin A from vitamin D was made by Harry Steenbock (1886–1967) in 1921. Vitamin E was first noted in 1923 by Herbert McLean Evans (1882–1972). Vitamin C was first isolated by Albert Szent-Gyorgyi (1893–   ). Vitamin K was discovered in 1929 by Henrik Dam (1895–   ). The separation of the various water-soluble vitamins originally called Vitamin B was started in 1928 by Robert R. Williams (1886–1965).

Knowledge of micronutrients has developed slowly. Iron was first directly used in the treatment of chlorotic anemia in 1832 by Pierre Blaud (1774–1858). The discovery of iodine as necessary in the functioning of the thyroid gland was made by Eugen Baumann (1846–1896) in 1895. Cobalt was found in 1948 to be an essential part of vitamin B_{12} by Edward Rickes (1912–   ). The nutritional importance of such micronutrients as zinc was only recently recognized.

On the other hand, fluorine's relationship to the prevention of dental caries, although a relatively recent finding, has excited a great deal of popular interest. This has resulted in public health measures for adding fluorine to drinking water in order to prevent dental caries.

Malnutrition is commonplace these days, not only in poverty-stricken areas but also in highly civilized communities where there is so much vogue for processed foods. Dr. Erwin Di Cyan has wisely indicated the extent of birth defects resulting from vitamin and micronutrient deficiencies.

This is a truly valuable book. It is carefully organized and the information in it is sound. Fortunately government regulations in the United States require full labeling of preparations for vitamin and mineral supplements. As Dr. Di Cyan says, one should read labels, carefully.

Dr. Di Cyan has thoughtfully added a helpful reading list for those who may be inspired to study recent reports on vitamins and minerals. The recommended daily allowance for vitamins and minerals is also wisely included.

Dr. Di Cyan's book is thus not merely a helpful, easily digested manual on vitamins and micronutrients, it is also a useful reference book. Current interest among our young people in "organic foods" makes Dr. Di Cyan's book particularly important. It gives the facts on which so much of the vogue for organic foods is based, and these facts can help to put the fad on an intellectually sound basis.

CHAUNCEY D. LEAKE, PH.D., SC.D.
School of Medicine
Department of Pharmacology
University of California at San Francisco

VITAMINS
IN YOUR LIFE

1

HOW BEST TO USE THIS BOOK

THE MOST DIFFICULT PART of writing a book dealing with facts is organizing it. What will you put where? The problem is not simply what to include but also what to omit to prevent an unintended side effect: putting the reader to sleep. The subject does not lend itself to easy solutions. One reason: there are sincere differences of opinion among experts. Since many conflicting opinions cannot be reconciled, I believed it was best to interpret them for the reader.

I organized this book in a fashion that I believe will most likely make it easiest for the reader to use. Therefore I have repeated certain aspects in relation to each of the vitamins and the micronutrients (trace minerals or trace elements). This should give the reader most of the information on a particular substance within one chapter, without excessive cross-reference. But vitamins and micronutrients, like people, are interdependent. Often they have more than one function or role. For that reason, too, do not zero in on one vitamin or micronutrient as if it were the royal remedy. There is no royal remedy or unitary solution due to the incredibly complex functions and interrelationships in man's metabolic machine.

Moreover I suggest that before you turn to the chapter on a

specific vitamin or micronutrient, you first read such explanatory chapters as "Vitamins as Sentinels" and "Enzymes: The Seven Dwarfs in the Cell Itself." Similarly, before you start a chapter on a particular trace mineral or micronutrient, turn to the general discussion "Micronutrients."

Except for rather important discoveries made before 1960 I refer to the literature of 1960 or later. That year is not a magic figure but it does encompass both material that is recent as well as earlier material that has been recently confirmed.

Finally, I invite your attention to the chapters at the back of the book dealing with some fundamental aspects of vitamins and micronutrients, as well as to the early chapter "Guide to the Concerned or Perplexed," which contains an overview and general discussion of food and nutrition and hopefully presents a framework that should enable you to interpret and put in a better focus the variety of information that often assails the reader in this perplexing field, where yesterday's superstition becomes today's dogma, and conversely, yesterday's facts become today's delusions.

E. D.

2

SOME DEFINITIONS

You will meet some probably unfamiliar terms in reading about vitamins, micronutrients and nutrition. For that reason let us define some of them at the outset.

A *vitamin* is a member of a group of chemicals or certain organic substances which have all of the following characteristics in common:

1. It is found in minute amounts in various foodstuffs.
2. It is indispensable in normal metabolism.
3. Its absence causes certain specific deficiency diseases which are serious and can be life-threatening.
4. Minute amounts often reverse the deficiency symptoms, though they do not usually repair the damage that had already taken place—as, for example, vitamin A will stop certain deficiency symptoms such as difficulty of vision in the dusk but does not cure blindness, which is a grave effect of long-continued vitamin A deficiency.
5. And as if that is not enough, a vitamin also functions as a coenzyme in an enzyme reaction.

A *coenzyme* is a nonprotein substance that works with or is bound to the protein part of an enzyme, which part is called an apoenzyme. The complete enzyme is called a holoenzyme and is composed of a coenzyme and apoenzyme. An enzyme does not work unless it is complete—hence, a coenzyme (a role that many vitamins, especially those of the B complex group, take) is necessary to its function. An example of a coenzyme is pantothenic acid.

An *enzyme* is a protein substance of highly complex structure that functions as a catalyst, hastening or enabling biological changes to take place. No living organism can exist without enzymes, which actually enable it to live by accelerating its biological or metabolic changes. (See Chapter 14, "Enzymes: The Seven Dwarfs in the Cell Itself.")

Species differences refers to the differences in response of different animals. The nutritional needs and metabolic equipment of all animals are not the same—hence different needs. For example, rats and other animals make their own vitamin C; man cannot and therefore must take it from outside. Most of our basic nutritional information is derived from work on rats. They were chosen because they are nearest to man in nutritional needs, and also cheaper as laboratory animals than monkeys; but it does not mean that information derived from animal feeding studies always applies to man. The best way to determine how a nutrient works in man is to study its effect in man. And even in man there are differences from individual to individual, i.e., biological variation within the same species. This applies to man as well as to other animals. Owing to inherited traits one individual may have greater need for a given vitamin or micronutrient than another.

Metabolism is a continuous process going on in the body which converts foodstuffs into energy or into other substances necessary to the functioning of the body. A *metabolite* is a product of metabolism; it may be an intermediate or an end product. Metabolites too are involved in normal functioning as some substances must first be converted into other substances (metabolites) before they can be utilized by the body. For example, thiamine (B_1) is not used by the body per se but is first converted into a metabolite called thiamine pyrophosphate. Consider metabolites like scrip, which must be converted into money before you can buy with it.

Micronutrients, or *trace minerals* or *trace metals,* so called because they are necessary in minute amounts or traces, are found largely in plants, in rocks of the earth's crust or in animals which in turn derive them from food or other sources in their environment. Some micronutrients appear to be necessary; others are known to be necessary or even critical in a variety of biochemical events that take place in metabolism. (The term *micronutrient* is used in this book to encompass trace minerals, trace metals and other trace elements.)

Antimetabolite is a word not frequently seen except in the scientific literature. An antimetabolite is a substance that antagonizes the action of a metabolite. It usually is similar to the metabolite it antagonizes, hence competes with it or may replace it in the metabolic scheme of things to the detriment of the body. For example, methionine, an amino acid, is a necessary metabolite; ethionine is its antimetabolite. At times an antimetabolite is used intentionally to interfere with a disease process, as methotrexate, an antimetabolite used in treating some forms of cancer.

An *antivitamin* is an antimetabolite against a vitamin which it replaces or competes with, to the detriment of the body. Deoxypyridoxine is an antimetabolite to pyridoxine (B_6); oxythiamine and pyrithiamine are antivitamins to thiamine (B_1).

Precursors are substances that are per se inactive but are converted in the body to a form that is active. For example, carotene, the yellow-orange-red coloring matter of vegetables, does not as such have vitamin A activity, but the body converts it into an active material that has vitamin A activity.

3

GUIDE TO THE CONCERNED OR PERPLEXED: GENERAL COMMENTS ABOUT FOOD AND NUTRITION

IN ASSESSING vitamin content of foods you cannot keep a ledger account. A rational way of keeping ahead of the game is to observe variety in your diet. Foods differ in vitamin and micronutrient content, and some foods, like whole wheat cereals, may inactivate a food micronutrient, and these are reasons, among others, that the supplementation of the diet by extra vitamins is desirable.

When buying vitamins you may well be seduced by attractive super-duper names, high-potency claims, etc. Such descriptions are not informative. What is informative in a vitamin and mineral capsule or tablet is the quantitative statement of the vitamins that *each* tablet or capsule contains. And check if the amount stated is per single tablet or capsule, because at times the quantities stated are per daily dose, and elsewhere on the label you may read that the daily dose is three tablets or capsules.

If you fail to grasp something it may not be your inadequate understanding. Nutrition, and especially its application, is not yet an exact science. Another reason is that the answer may not be known. Still another problem enters: often there are conflicting opinions among authorities who hold different views, due either to their own experience which may differ from others', or to a differing interpretation of the facts that have been developed or observed.

Essential

The word *essential* is often used in connection with nutrition. It has the usual connotation except that in nutrition it also means that a certain substance is necessary to avoid deficiency symptoms which can produce severe illness, not just necessary for comfort.

In connection with amino acids, the word *essential* has an additional meaning. Other amino acids, in addition to those termed essential, are just as necessary, but since they can be manufactured by the body (often at the expense of other substances), they are not labeled essential. The essential amino acids are as follows:

Isoleucine	Leucine	Lysine
Methionine	Cystine	Phenylalanine
Tyrosine	Threonine	Tryptophan
Valine		

Food Selection

Good nutrition is not a fixation on vitamins, minerals or micronutrients, lecithin, vegetables, fruits or any other single stuff, but a combination of foods. Some vitamins require other foodstuffs for absorption or utilization. Think in terms of *food*, supplemented by vitamins and micronutrients.

Food serves purposes in addition to nutrition; namely, it lends a feeling of comfort, body warmth, and even security. It also represents power among groups of people as nations.

One of the causes of malnutrition—which can also mean an unbalanced food intake, not just an insufficient one—is devotion to dislikes, which may have originated in childhood, or to ethnic food habits. They are usually not rational and often they militate against optimal nutrition either through (a) avoiding a desirable food, (b) overbalancing with other food substances, or (c) retaining taboos. Avoid such habits and dislikes if they do not serve you well nutritionally and if you can reason with your emotions, which is more easily said than done. For example, there is no rational reason for avoiding horsemeat; in the United States people have not developed a taste for it and it is tagged with the opprobrium that only poor people eat it. Fifty years ago liver was also tagged as a poor man's meat. The societal sanction against it dissolved when it was discovered that it controls pernicious anemia, a hitherto fatal disease.

Good nutrition also requires water. It serves more than to satisfy thirst. It is necessary for a medium of energy conversion because the biochemical events that produce energy take place in an aqueous medium. Severe curtailment of water may produce a dehydration which can be a serious condition. Water also serves as a waste-disposal medium; for example, uric acid, a waste product, is disposed of in an aqueous medium by being washed out by the kidneys through the urine.

Diets

In their attempt at reducing body weight people often go on a distorted diet. Many are indeed successful—body weight is reduced. But the matter is far from complete with the loss of weight. Here are only a few reasons why you must look further when you plan reducing body weight:

1. Some regimens reduce only water, not fat. This is the principal reason for weight reduction that stops after an initial loss.
2. Some diets largely reduce muscle rather than fat. This can be harmful, especially in older people.
3. High-protein diets with only a minimum of carbohydrates do indeed reduce weight. However, kidney function can be damaged and a uric acid accumulation may produce kidney stones; in addition a rise in the cholesterol level in the blood from the almost exclusive use of protein and fat, without adequate carbohydrate, can result.
4. The problem in reducing does not lie in the initial taking off of weight, but in retaining the lower weight, which is most difficult without adherence to wise eating habits.
5. Emphasizing proteins at the expense of other food elements is unwise, because the others are equally necessary for adequate functioning of the body. For example, fat is an energy reserve or depot and most efficient for energy production. Sugar, i.e., glucose, conserves protein. Hence, avoiding any trace of sugar which is converted to glucose serves the body ill because this protein-sparing effect is lost. The protein content in the body is comparatively smaller than that of fat or carbohydrate and is necessary for many biochemical events that take place.
6. High-protein, low-carbohydrate diets have another drawback, according to the nutrition studies done by Dr. Harold Yacowitz of the Health Research Institute of Fairleigh Dickinson University. While the overweight people in the study did lose weight, laboratory determinations done on them showed a breakdown of tissue protein despite the high-protein diet, and an increase in the excretion of calcium, phosphorus, and the micronutrients iron and zinc. These findings show a loss of bone substance as well as that of protein.

See Chapter 19, "Obesity," for a comprehensive discussion of weight reduction.

Alcohol

Throughout this book reference is made to the dire things that befall alcoholics, how they deprive themselves of vitamins, micronutrients, and generally raise nutritional havoc with themselves. The mistaken idea is still current that alcoholics are found on skid row. While that is true, they are also found in executive suites, homes, everywhere, often holding positions of responsibility. How they discharge their responsibilities is another matter—alcohol is usually a good solvent for sound judgment.

One must not give precedence to labels over meanings. Few, if any, will admit they are alcoholics—a term that has different meanings to different people. Some maintain that one cannot be an alcoholic unless one drinks alone, which is untrue. Considerable and regular indulgence in alcohol carries the nutritional stigmata of alcoholism no matter what the label.

But alcohol—which is probably our number-one drug problem —has the approbation of society and has societal sanction for festive occasions. I do not mean that an occasional drink will wipe out your vitamins and micronutrients. Its damage may be infinitesimal and there is no ruler against which this can be measured. Nonetheless, infinitesimal damage grows with addition and attrition. Beyond this, it is not possible to set the amounts of alcohol that one should or should not drink.

Yet, the effect of alcohol goes farther than depletion of vitamins and micronutrients. You may not be aware that there is a clear relationship between cholesterol and alcohol. People cut down their dietary intake of eggs and other animal foods in order to reduce the amount of cholesterol they ingest. For example, they will use polyunsaturated fats and avoid butter, but at the same meal they will have cocktails or other alcoholic drinks, forgetting that alcohol increases cholesterol in the body.

Not that alcohol contains cholesterol—it does not. But even a moderate amount of alcohol increases stores in the body or in the circulation of plasma triglycerides. These are similar to cholesterol; both are part of what is called the lipoprotein molecule. In fact, there is increasing evidence that the triglycerides may have an even more important role in association with heart attack than cholesterol. (Carbohydrates also increase these triglycerides.)

When alcohol is taken in larger than moderate quantities a dramatic thing can happen: not only are the triglycerides steeply increased but the cholesterol level in the blood can rise to heights far in excess of what may be imagined on a cholesterol-rich diet.

Milk

Milk is a fine, though *not* the perfect food—there are no unitary perfect foods. However, since it is one of the basic and most widely used foods, the following listing of vitamins and micronutrients should be helpful in assessing its advantages and deficiencies.

Depending on the season of year and other variable factors, the listed vitamins in milk will vary. The amounts shown represent average figures accepted by most nutrition authorities.

The milk customarily sold (called whole milk) contains 3.25 to 3.75 percent butterfat. The fat content of milk from Jersey cows is almost 5 percent. One quart of such milk is equivalent to about 650 calories, depending on the fat content. Thus a glassful of milk is equivalent to 160 calories. Whole milk contains about 140 mg cholesterol per quart, or 35 mg per glassful, or 70 mg per pint.

Vitamins in Milk
per pint (2 glasses)

Vitamin A	346–420 IU	⎫
Vitamin D	400 IU (when fortified)	
Vitamin E	34–854 mcg	fat-soluble
Vitamin K	Trace	⎭
Vitamin B_1	0.15 mg	⎫
Vitamin B_2	0.82 mg	
Vitamin B_6	0.23 mg	
Vitamin B_{12}	0.64 mcg	
Biotin	16.55 mcg	water-soluble
Folacin	1.09 mcg	
Niacin	0.49 mg	
Pantothenic acid	1.66 mg	
Vitamin C	4.88 mg	⎭

Micronutrients in Milk

	Estimated Daily Requirement for Adults	Amount in Milk mg per pint (2 glasses)
Cobalt	3–5 mcg B_{12}	2.64 mcg B_{12}
Copper	2 mg	0.14 mg
Fluorine		0.75 mcg
Iodine	100–150 mcg	0.10 mcg
Iron	See inside front cover	0.46 mg
Magnesium	200–400 mg	60 mg
Manganese	3–9 mg	0.009 mg
Molybdenum		0.03 mg
Zinc	10–15 mg	1.80 mg

Adapted from *National Dairy Council Digest*, 39:26, 1968.

A reduced-fat milk contains 2 percent butterfat. This is equivalent to 140 calories per glassful. The difference is small. Thus the caloric "bargain" of the so-called low-fat 2 percent milk is deceptive.

However, nonfat dry milk, when reconstituted with water, is an excellent product for a number of reasons. First, it yields only about half the number of calories of whole milk, namely 325 calories per quart. Second, the calories are derived from the protein and carbohydrate content, not the fat. But since the fat is abstracted from nonfat milk, it contains no fat-soluble vitamins —A, D and E. However, most nonfat dry milk is fortified with vitamins A and D, but not with E.

Milk is a poor source of iron and vitamin C, which should be supplemented from other sources.

People with high blood pressure or others who should restrict their intake of salt should bear in mind that milk is relatively high in salt, containing about 500 mg per quart. A low-sodium milk which contains only a relatively small amount of sodium (about 25 mg per quart) is obtainable.

Milk Intolerance. While milk is a splendid though incomplete food there is a phenomenon called *lactose intolerance* which should be noted. Lactose intolerance means that the individual who has it does not respond well to lactose. Our ordinary table sugar is sucrose; the natural sugar in milk is lactose. The reason for lactose intolerance on the part of some people is not allergy to milk, but the lack of, or more frequently a low level of, a certain enzyme, called *lactase,* which metabolizes or hydrolyzes lactose. (Enzymes usually end in *ase;* sugars usually end in *ose.*)

People who respond adversely to lactose or milk sugar usually have a low level of intestinal lac*tase,* but they may have no other digestive anomalies. The condition is most frequent in the genetic stock in the vicinity of the Mediterranean—more particularly, in Greeks, Jews, Arabs and Africans, although a fair proportion of Japanese and Filipinos are also reported to have a low lactase level. It is infrequent among western Europeans and Scandinavian people. Low levels of lactase may well be a quite normal occurrence, because in most animals, the lactase level normally falls after weaning.

What happens if you have lactose intolerance or a low level of lactase and you drink milk? Nothing grave but something quite uncomfortable. Cramps and diarrhea may occur or the only symptoms may be gas and a bloated feeling. Yet, people who have a low level of lactase may be able to drink a fair amount of milk without discomfort provided that they consume it with meals. They should also avoid drinking ice-cold milk, especially in large amounts. But they may be able to tolerate milk products, as cheese, buttermilk or yogurt. The best test is individual trial to determine what milk products in what amounts are tolerated without discomfort. Children may develop such milk intolerance as they mature, although many of them had had no discomfort after drinking milk as children.

Should You Take Supplements?

It will be pointed out throughout this book that vitamins, minerals, micronutrients do not take the place of food. It's probable that a carefully balanced diet will give you sufficient quantities of each. But for a number of reasons, people often eat as they conveniently choose, without careful attention to diet. To make sure that your intake of vitamins and micronutrients is adequate, supplements are available. But, again, do not take them in place of food, but in addition to a well-balanced diet.

How will you be able to evaluate foods? By reference to nutritional information, indeed, but also by thoughtful reading of the labels on processed foods. For example, boxed cereals usually do have a moderate quantity of these food elements—vitamins and minerals. But you cannot be certain unless you thoughtfully *read the labels*. In doing so, you may well be able to compare them with other foodstuffs and will be able to make an intelligent evaluation.

4

WHY VITAMINS?

Do you need vitamins and minerals? No one disputes that you cannot live without them—though you need more than vitamins and minerals to live. Vitamins are not a substitute for good nutrition.

Many doctors say that you don't need extra vitamins, that you get all that you ordinarily need in a good American diet. But what is a good diet? Is there such a thing as the American diet? Who observes it and uses it? Can you get enough vitamins and micronutrients from your food? The answer to that is *yes* and *no*.

There are many reasons why one cannot depend upon the so-called good American diet to get a sufficient amount and variety of vitamins and micronutrients, despite the fact that most food-stuffs contain them, and here are some of them:

1. The vitamins in the food may suffer a deterioration by the method of food preparation. Also, some vitamins and micronutrients may be discarded in the cooking water used in the preparation of the food. Garbage can thus become nutritious.
2. People often dislike foods that are good for them. Since people do not readily eat food they hate, it is next to impossible to recommend a standard diet that is realistic.

3. Certain ethnic groups will not eat some of the American or other staples—for example, Oriental people prefer rice as their staple carbohydrate. Moreover, many ethnic diets are clearly overbalanced in certain food elements and rather short in others. The Italian diet is a case in point, being heavy in carbohydrates and fat.
4. The commercial processing of food, as well as its storage, often reduces the vitamin content. This is particularly true of vitamin E.
5. People living on small pensions which are further reduced in buying power by inflation cannot afford to buy the foods that may be recommended as sources of good nutrition. This may well apply to people living on welfare or in poverty pockets. Whether they can afford supplementary vitamins is another question.
6. Older people have their dietary preferences or rigidities and are more at home with the old superstitions as to foods and food mixtures than with the so-called American diet. Regional preferences are also strongly entrenched.
7. Stable amounts of vitamins and minerals are often largely dependent on geographical and climatological differences which make the so-called American diet a myth.
8. The recognition that reliance cannot be put on the American diet as a dependable source of vitamins and micronutrients was the motivating factor behind the food enrichment programs, in which specific amounts of vitamins, as niacin or iron, are added to certain foods.
9. Seasonal variations in foods prevent reliance on foods solely as a source of vitamins. For example, annually there is a striking eightfold difference in the content of vitamin E in milk—the least in the spring and the most in the fall. Yet, Vitamin E deficiency is unknown in adults.

All these reasons speak for the wisdom of adequate supplementation of vitamins and minerals as well as micronutrients in the diet.

Vitamins, minerals and micronutrients are not something apart from living and good health. Conversely, alone they are not enough; they are merely part of, though an irreplaceable part of, an overall diet. A balance of other elements, proteins, carbohydrates and fats, is also needed for good physical and mental functioning of the organism. As a matter of fact, the relationship of vitamins, minerals and micronutrients to other food substances is so interdependent that both food and supplemental vitamins are needed for optimum nutrition.

Deficiencies

When deficiencies occur they are usually multiple, i.e., deficiencies in more than one vitamin, mineral or micronutrient. These are usually a result of inadequate food habits. No Biblical manna answers the need for optimum nutrition.

There are many reasons why deficiencies in vitamins, minerals or micronutrients can arise. Here are some of them:

1. Malabsorption: when there is a functional impediment to absorption in the small intestine, vitamins or minerals cannot be utilized, though they may be in food or supplemental intake in sufficient amounts. This applies principally to the fat-soluble vitamins—A, D, E and K.
2. Deficiency can arise through an insufficient intake. This may occur through highly restricted diets or when an individual is on a starvation level of food intake. Older people, especially those living alone, often have vitamin and micronutrient deficiencies as they will not prepare food for themselves but instead live on toast, jam and tea.
3. A metabolic impediment (aside from the ordinary fat malabsorption) may prevent the conversion to an active form of a vitamin, though enough of a vitamin precursor is taken in—as failure to convert carotene, a

precursor to active vitamin A, may produce vitamin A deficiency.

4. Excessive intake of other food substances may make an otherwise adequate amount of vitamin insufficient—for example, a high carbohydrate intake increases the requirement for B_1.

5. Certain disease conditions increase the need for a given vitamin—for example, high thyroid activity with its higher metabolic activity also increases the need for thiamine, or vitamin B_1.

6. An increased consumption at the expense of a more balanced diet—as, for example, people who *drink* their lunch or dinner at the expense of eating, creating alcoholic malnutrition.

7. A stepped-up destruction or excretion of a vitamin—as, for example, when increased urination takes place as a result of therapy with diuretics; therewith, an increased amount of water-soluble vitamins, minerals or micronutrients is excreted.

8. Anomalous distribution of a vitamin or mineral in the body—as, for example, in liver disease, fat-soluble vitamins may not be adequately stored in the liver.

9. Advent of stress—for example, in tissue injury the need for certain vitamins, minerals and micronutrients may be greatly increased. There is increased stress in infections— viral or bacterial—or in an unusual environment as met by astronauts and, conversely, by divers.

10. Normally increased tissue requirements—as in growth or adolescence or in pregnancy the need for nutrients including vitamins, minerals and micronutrients is increased. If the need is not met, a mild or moderate deficiency may occur.

These are only some of the reasons deficiencies of various degrees can occur. There are other causes as well, as if these were not enough. The objective should be to provide sufficient vitamins, minerals and micronutrients before damage is done.

When there is a high alcoholic intake or even often in so-called social drinking a high intake of vitamins is especially desirable because of the extensive, often hidden, damage done by alcohol. The greater intake of vitamins is necessary because vitamins B_1, B_6 and biotin are necessary to support the oxidation-inducing enzymes; nicotinic acid and B_2 are needed to overcome the inhibition of metabolic conversions caused by alcohol; vitamin E to prevent the increased peroxidation of fats in the liver; more folic acid, vitamins B_6 and B_{12} to repair the tissue damage that alcohol produces; and vitamin C to keep connective tissue in healthy condition. The whole principle is one of *repair and replacement*—the repair of tissues (when possible) and the replacement of the vitamins either excreted or not taken in food. Increased urination during drinking also can deplete minerals, which should be replaced through food.

These are some of the reasons why it may be well to assure an adequate intake of vitamins and minerals by taking daily vitamin and micronutrient supplements.

There are a number of other problems in obtaining sufficient vitamins, minerals or micronutrients. One of them is an upset of the vitamin balance when large quantities of one vitamin are taken to the exclusion of others. Another has to do with antibiotics. Some antibiotics increase the need for riboflavin, or vitamin B_2, as they reduce either the body stores or methods of utilization of the vitamin. Or a change in the kind and balance of bacteria normally found in the intestine induced by antibiotics can produce a distortion in the balance of vitamins. For example, vitamin K is normally synthesized in the intestine, and an intestinal upset can inhibit the body synthesis of vitamin K. If that is extreme it can lead to bleeding, such as the appearance of small hemorrhages in the skin.

When we say that we, as people, require vitamins it is because certain functions in the body require them. For example, our life, largely though not exclusively, is a matter of enzyme function. An enzyme is mainly a catalyst. (See Chapter 14 on enzymes and Chapter 3 for more details.) Each little biochemical reaction in the body has its own enzyme—and there are thousands of reactions, hence thousands of different enzymes performing the physiological task of living. For example, an enzyme, *serum transaminase* (an indicator of heart action), requires sufficient vitamin B_6 for its function. Similarly, another enzyme, *red blood cell transketolase*, must have sufficient B_1 to exert its activity in blood metabolism.

The traffic signs that direct the function of the vitamins and micronutrients in the body are not clear; many misdirections can therefore occur. If all goes according to schedule, then all is well. But let there be a slight mixup in the traffic signals and anything can happen. The individual who harbors such a traffic mixup can give signs of deficiency even though he takes enough of a given vitamin to prevent a deficiency.

For example, there is an amino acid called *tryptophan*. It plays a role in the production of many vital substances and is much sought after in the body as an ingredient in or component of several biochemical transactions. Sometimes, an unlooked-for reaction occurs in the body, as in a certain cancerlike condition called carcinoid. This cancerlike condition makes serotonin —a useful substance for other purposes—and when the carcinoid is avid for serotonin, it uses up all the tryptophan it can get to make the serotonin.

Tryptophan is also necessary, in fact indispensable, in another biochemical transaction, i.e., for the smooth functioning of the nicotinic acid cycle. But if the tryptophan is used up by the cancerlike carcinoid, there is no tryptophan left to use in the nicotinic acid cycle and a deficiency may occur. That is one example where a deficiency of a vitamin can occur (in this instance, nicotinic acid) when one of the members of the natural convoy (tryptophan) for the production of nicotinic acid is lacking. One of the symptoms of nicotinic acid deficiency is pellagra, with its mental and skin symptoms.

Such a situation as just described is now rare and if it occurs it is not for self-treatment. You cannot cure it just by taking nicotinic acid. It is given here as an oversimplified example of the competition for vital metabolites or substances that continually goes on in the body and which often requires more than the minimum recommended amount of a vitamin.

How much vitamin, mineral or micronutrient is enough? To answer that question two tables—the Recommended Daily Allowances (RDA) and the U.S. Recommended Daily Allowances (U.S. RDA)—have been promulgated, which are believed to be sufficient to prevent deficiency for the average person in good health. They do not refer to the amounts needed in certain stresses (except pregnancy). (Moreover, Dr. Linus Pauling and Dr. Roger Williams have postulated that in many individuals the constitutional need may be ten or more times the recommended daily allowances.)

U.S. RDA and RDA

RDA stands for Recommended Daily Allowances.

The U.S. RDA are legal definitions controlled by the Food and Drug Administration (FDA), and will be found on the outside of the back cover. They are adaptations from the RDA promulgated by the National Academy of Sciences–National Research Council (NAS–NRC), which will be found on the insides of both covers.

Vitamin products are labeled under the U.S. RDA, which have

the force of law. By and large they are sound and should guard you against deficiencies unless you have an increased need over and above the amounts listed.

Fortunately, views change with the availability of new information. For example, vitamin E was at one time not recognized to be useful in *human* nutrition (emphasis is on *human* as it was long recognized as necessary in the nutriture of other animals). But now the RDA include vitamin E as necessary and state the amounts in different age groups.

In 1966, the Food and Nutrition Board of the National Research Council, which, while it does not have the force of law, has the respect and confidence of the scientific world, clearly promulgated its decision that vitamin E is necessary for human nutrition and well-being and stated the amount necessary for that purpose, working out a schedule. That schedule is part of the RDA found on the inside of both covers of this book. This was taken into the U.S. RDA, found on the outside back cover.

I am aware that the difference between the U.S. RDA and the RDA of the NAS–NRC can be confusing. But you can simplify the situation and derive meaningful information by considering the U.S. RDA to be legal definitions under which vitamin and mineral products are labeled, and the RDA of the NAS–NRC to be more extensive in its information.

These are not magic figures and the amount of any vitamins and minerals can well be, and has been, periodically revised up or down. This is fortunate, as we are in a land that has huge areas of ignorance in nutrition, as well as in some other disciplines. Indeed what we need is vitamins, minerals and micronutrients, but what we need more is additional research. That is intellectual nutrition.

5

THE SKIN VITAMIN—VITAMIN A

THE EARLIEST VITAMIN discovered, vitamin A, often called the skin vitamin, can just as well be called the hair vitamin, or eye and sight vitamin, the glandular, or teeth and gums vitamin, since it has a profound effect upon the development and well-being of all these structures. It also plays a role in resistance to infection, hence is also an antiinfection vitamin. It is involved as well in the health of the mucous membranes lining the respiratory and the digestive tract—in fact, in the top layer, called the epithelium, of most inner structures of the body as well as the external skin we show the world. When there is a deficiency of vitamin A the skin takes on a dryness, with raised little goosefleshlike bumps.

This vitamin takes on a double importance in children, since it deals with their development and presages what the adult's health may be. Yet there is a substantial deficiency of vitamin A in many parts of the world.

Deficiency

Why would there be a deficiency of vitamin A during our *advanced* state of technology, especially when vitamin A is plentiful in foods and huge quantities are synthetically produced?

At the third Western Hemisphere Nutrition Congress in 1971 sponsored by the American Medical Association and American Institute of Nutrition, Robert E. Hodges, professor of medicine at the University of California at Davis, made a sage observation: that estimates of the need for vitamin A by people in general have been based upon samples of populations that are usually well-fed and do not have signs of vitamin A deficiency, upon populations poorly fed which do have signs of such deficiency and upon amounts required by animals. Extrapolating these observations, it has been concluded that there is a greater vitamin A deficiency than generally was believed to exist.

This is exactly what was reported at the same congress by T. Keith Murray, Ph.D., Chief of the Nutrition Research Division of Canada's Food and Drug Directorates:

> A significant percentage of most age groups in North America lack appreciable liver reserves of vitamin A, and 20 to 30 percent fail to consume the recommended daily allowances. And although most North American adults have adequate blood levels of vitamin A, an important number of children fall below the acceptable level, with adverse health effects to some of them.

At an earlier meeting, the second Western Hemisphere Nutrition Congress held in Puerto Rico in 1968, Dr. Murray also reported a "shocking" incidence of vitamin A deficiency in Canada, and even at that time believed that the same might very well apply to the United States. That the dietary intake of vitamin A may not account for the whole story was Dr. Murray's belief. Poor absorption and other factors were being investigated to determine if they have a role in such widespread deficiency.

Do not run to the nearest friendly corner drugstore to load up on vitamin A as the remedy for all your troubles because the story is more complex than that, and requires highly astute scientific detective work to get to the meaning of vitamin A deficiency. The reason is a nasty little fact that crept into Murray's work— namely, a small proportion of human livers assayed at autopsy for vitamin A showed no liver stores *at all,* yet the people had not shown any signs of vitamin A deficiency.

We will go into this topic later in this chapter. But vitamin A deficiency is nearer home than we think. In New York City, in children 12 years old and younger, low vitamin A levels are said to be quite common, and poor children, i.e., those of low-income families, had about three times the frequency of low vitamin A levels of the more economically advantaged.

While this is a small sample, it strongly suggests that inadequate nutrition is economic. However, economics alone is not the cause for poor nutrition. A number of variables enter, one of which is the educational level of the parents, as well as ethnic food habits. You do not eat the food that is *good for you* if you are unaccustomed to it.

To check if this reasoning applies, let us look at a small part of the imposing 1968–1970 Ten-State National Nutrition Survey, authorized by Congress in 1967. This was originally headed by Arnold E. Schaefer, Ph.D., Chief of the Nutrition Program of the Center for Disease Control. Owing to political considerations, Dr. Schaefer terminated his connection with the study near the end of the program. It was subsequently edited and published in five volumes in 1972 by the Department of Health, Education and Welfare.

The study reports that in the low-income states there is a severe vitamin A deficiency in all ages of the Spanish-American population and only a minimal deficiency in the high-income states in the Spanish-American and other populations. The low-income states are Kentucky, Louisiana, South Carolina, Texas and West Virginia. The high-income states are California, Massachusetts, Michigan, New York and Washington. In short, vitamin A deficiency is due probably to economic and educational factors, as well as to ethnic food practices.

What Does Deficiency Really Mean?

You must distinguish among deficiencies because the word is used in more than one context. One deficiency means that there is a lower than desirable amount, or none, of a given vitamin in a foodstuff, i.e., the *foodstuff* is broadly said to be *deficient* in it. For example, raisins are deficient in vitamin A, so are most breadstuffs.

Deficiency also means that not enough of a given vitamin is in a whole daily diet, and therefore the *intake* is deficient. For example, alcoholics are usually deficient in vitamin A (and other vitamins, especially those of the B complex group) because their food intake is low. People who vigorously avoid fats in their food and do not take a supplement of vitamin A will also have a deficient intake.

A third deficiency means that a doctor finds that the blood level of a given vitamin is lower than the range customarily found in people. More precisely, the person may not be deficient but merely has a low level of a given vitamin in the blood.

Deficiency is also used in a fourth sense, namely, when certain manifestations are said to be symptoms of vitamin deficiency. For example, when a doctor sees an individual who complains of dry mouth, nostrils and throat, has poor vision in the dusk or in other dim light, has lusterless eyes, irritated eyelids, and dry, scaly skin, raised bumps like goose pimples, he may suspect that the individual has a vitamin A deficiency. Not all of the possible signs or symptoms of vitamin A deficiency appear at one time, nor do signs of deficiency suddenly occur.

And an individual may have had his vitamin A stores depleted and not show signs of deficiency for a long time. In fact, he may not be deficient in vitamin A at all if you consider a fifth meaning of deficiency: he may have an adequate store of vitamin A in the liver, but because of a liver or other dysfunction he *does not mobilize* it from the liver into the tissues.

A sixth form of deficiency: an individual may have a good and adequate daily intake of vitamin A and yet does not absorb it, due to a condition called *malabsorption* in which there is poor absorption of fats. Malabsorption is an intestinal dysfunction which may have one of a number of causes. Vitamin A requires fat for its absorption. Such people excrete the fat they take in their food (steatorrhea), one of the causes of which may be an inability to secrete enough bile acids or bile salts from the gallbladder which emulsify the fats and facilitate absorption through the intestinal walls. Such people require vitamin A by injections (as well as other fat-soluble vitamins, that is, D, E, K) which a physician administers.

Signs of Deficiency

What can happen if you do not take enough vitamin A in food or as a supplement? Many things—all of them bad. At first, nothing happens that is apparent. But in young children, those younger than six years, deficiency can eventually lead to blindness. This is an extreme result and not found in the United States as far as we know. Infection and ulceration of the eye can develop before blindness occurs.

At all ages one of the early signs of vitamin A deficiency is inability to adapt vision in semidarkness (night blindness), a lackluster appearance of the eyeball which loses its normal glistening look due to dryness (xerophthalmia), as well as scaly and dry appearance of the eyelids.

Vitamin A is called the eye vitamin as well because vision itself depends on it. A chemical change takes place in the rods and cones structure of the eye in the absence of vitamin A which leads to blindness. In fact, *retinene,* a chemical vitamin A variant, is actually present in the fantastically complex structure of the eye.

The drying and hardening effect of the tissue of the eye and eyelid is based upon the need for vitamin A to assure the integrity of the epithelium. The epithelium is a most interesting structure—skin and not skin, call it a soft armor. It is the topmost layer of cells on the skin; it is also the topmost layer of cells on all other membranes—like mucous and serous membranes—and all surfaces inside and outside of the body. Inside of the body the epithelium, a microscopic layer of certain specialized cells, covers the glands, intestines, eyes, ears, respiratory tract, gums —in fact all surfaces. Outside the body the epithelial layer covers the skin with microscopically small cells, only a few layers thick—small enough to escape seeing with the naked eye. There are variants of epithelial cells on different organs which are adapted for different functions. For example, the epithelial cells on the outer skin are tougher than those that cover the membranes of the respiratory system, i.e., the bronchial tubes and lungs, and of the genitourinary tract.

Vitamin A assures the wholeness of the epithelium. The epithelium has a protective function against infection or other mishaps. That is the reason why in vitamin A deficiency, the integrity of the epithelium is damaged and infection can more easily occur. When that takes place, the result is seen in lusterless eyes, and the dry, lusterless inside of the bottom eyelids—xerophthalmia. The prefix *xeros* means dry.

Infections reduce the blood level of vitamin A. Hence, infections per se, whether they are from the common cold or other causes, create an increased need for vitamin A. They reduce the stores of vitamin A where we need it most, particularly for the integrity of the epithelium and for certain other lesser reasons.

A deficiency of vitamin A may create another skin change—a typical hardening of the skin, producing dryness and itching. At times, the hair follicles can become involved. In extreme cases, the skin takes on an appearance of goose pimples—hard, minute bumps on the skin which give it a feel of roughness as if one had been stroking a rasp. These bumps may become dark and resemble minute polka-dots where the hair follicles are.

Acne is of considerable concern to adolescents who have it. Its potential for scarring skin can leave an analogue—psychological scarring in boys and more particularly in girls. Vitamin A is no cureall for acne. Yet, the peer pressure for keeping down weight —often to the point of underweight—has adolescents substituting cola drinks for milk. (Two other reasons: milk is often considered "babyish" and "good-for-you"—two potent reasons for avoiding it.) Cola contains no vitamin A; milk is a rich source of it. It is wise to be assured that the teenager does have a reliable intake of vitamin A daily to retain the integrity of the epithelium as a help against acne. But bear in mind, acne is associated with the endocrinological upheaval of puberty. It is not a local skin disease.

Recently, vitamin A acid called *trans*-retinoic acid has been used by dermatologists as an aid in the treatment of acne. While it is quite effective, whether to use it must, however, be the decision of your dermatologist—not the teenager—as vitamin A acid is a skin irritant. In fact, the acne becomes worse during the first few weeks of treatment before improvement occurs.

An extension of the epithelium-saving effect of vitamin A is its effect upon the formation and growth of teeth. Both development of the teeth and the health of the gums during maturity are adversely affected if the integrity of the epithelium is impeded because of vitamin A deficiency.

Vitamin A deficiency can also interfere with the function of the glands that secrete hormones. This includes both the development of the reproductive system and its normal function when maturity has been reached. An important organ in the endocrinological orchestra involved is the adrenal gland. It has been reported that in vitamin A deficiency there is a reduced ability of the adrenal to secrete cortisone. The adrenal also secretes hormones other than cortisone, which emphasizes the importance of the role of vitamin A in the endocrine system.

The word *resistance* is used broadly and is used to express different concepts. If we consider resistance to infection to be aided by an intact epithelium, vitamin A is indeed a factor in resistance to infection. Obviously, it does not offer such resistance in an animal that is deficient in vitamin A. When we speak of resistance generally, we open a considerable discussion because resistance plays one of the most ubiquitous roles in disease and in health.

The property of vitamin A as an epithelializing vitamin comes to the fore in the healing of wounds. We have seen the relationship of vitamin A to the adrenals; there is a reduced ability of adrenal glands to secrete its hormone, cortisone, when there is a vitamin A deficiency. There is another side to this observation: the use of vitamin A facilitates wound healing where the healing is impeded by the individual's taking cortisone. Cortisone retards the healing of wounds. Dr. Thomas K. Hunt of the University of California at San Francisco used vitamin A on such wounds and was able to effect healing though the patients continued taking cortisone. Nonhealing wounds invite infection.

Bear in mind that even in the presence of the classic signs of vitamin A deficiency—such as xerophthalmia, night blindness, or the goose-pimpled skin—there may be other reasons for these symptoms. The recognition of the true deficiency requires diagnostic acumen, in addition to the use of laboratory gadgetry. In other words, when a determination of the vitamin A level in blood shows that level to be lower than that considered normal, it does not necessarily mean that the troubles all stem from deficiency of vitamin A. The symptoms may be due to another condition, quite unrelated or in addition to a low vitamin A level.

The thrust of this section is that while vitamin A is one of the most important vitamins—and every vitamin is important—do not jump to a conclusion.

How Does Deficiency Arise?

It is commonly believed that deficiency of vitamin A is due to eating a diet poor in vitamin A. That is true. But that is not the complete story because other events may also produce a deficiency. For example, infection depletes vitamin A stores in the body. With a chronic infection—genitourinary, respiratory or other that is long-continued—or when the loss of vitamin A becomes greater than the intake, infection can deplete the vitamin at a faster rate than the input from the daily diet.

Another reason for the loss or depletion of vitamin A may be liver disease, which interferes with the storage of the vitamin, or a reduced absorption because there is a malabsorption of fats. Absorption may also be impeded by a restricted diet because protein, as well as fat, is necessary for the absorption of vitamin A and its utilization by the body.

Failure to absorb vitamin A from food may occur if mineral oil is taken regularly to overcome constipation. It blocks the absorption of all fat-soluble vitamins, including vitamins A, D, E and K.

Perhaps a more frequent reason for vitamin A deficiency than we surmise is the inability of the body to convert carotene to a form of vitamin A used by it. (Carotene is a provitamin—a precursor for the body production of vitamin A.) This condition is often due to the lack of a converting enzyme. Beta-carotene is the yellow-orange pigment from vegetables.

When a deficiency has occurred how does one correct it? Usually deficiency can be corrected with only little residual damage, but not invariably. The eyes are most vulnerable to deficiency, and often the best hope is to arrest the damage that has occurred and to prevent it from progressing. Blindness is *not* reversible.

In countries with substantial vitamin A deprivation total blindness is not uncommon in children. During the Middle Ages there were many blind beggars; quite likely they were blind from childhood due to vitamin A deficiency.

Many symptoms of deficiency can be reversed or corrected by a continuing diet rich in vitamin A. At other times the use of vitamin A supplements—capsules, tablets, drops or even injections—may be advisable or even necessary. Do not diagnose your own fancied vitamin A deficiency. It requires the thoughtful attention of a nutritionally informed physician. Your problem may not be vitamin A deficiency. Better work on prevention through an adequate diet.

Vitamin A Poisoning

The expression "If a little bit is good a lot is better" is intended to be humorous but poisoning is not a joke. Vitamin A is one vitamin (vitamin D is another) where doses considerably larger than recommended have a potential for harm—and in extreme cases can poison the user.

For example, an 18-year-old girl was admitted to a hospital as an emergency due to symptoms of psychosis. She was depressed and agitated, and other symptoms suggested the tentative diagnosis of brain tumor. While under further observation in the hospital she improved spontaneously. It then developed that she had been taking 100,000 to 150,000 IU of vitamin A daily for months (20 to 30 times the RDA) for the treatment of her acne. After two weeks in the hospital during which she received no vitamin A, her condition became normal.

Mothers tend to overdose infants at times, in their enthusiasm, by giving several times the dose of vitamin A recommended. But poisoning with vitamin A is not often reported.

The symptoms of vitamin A poisoning vary. Sometimes there are restlessness, loss of appetite, loss of weight and hair, swelling over the long bones, muscle pains; or there may be liver or nervous disturbances. The treatment is to stop taking vitamin A.

Poisoning from vitamin A has also been reported from eating liver of polar bear, which is extremely rich in vitamin A, or even bear meat. The bear accumulates a tremendous amount of vitamin A to enable him to survive the many months of his hibernation. Depending on the time when he is killed, his flesh may be excessively rich in vitamin A—highest during the early part of his hibernation and lowest toward the end of the period.

What Is Vitamin A?

There are many types of vitamin A, all of which serve the same purposes. Some of the vitamin A-like substances are carotenes—the yellow-to-red pigments in vegetables. These carotenes are called provitamins A, because they are converted to the form of vitamin A the body uses. Other carotenes are used in coloring foods. In certain instances rats cannot convert carotene to vitamin A, but it is not known if that disability also applies to man.

Vitamin A is one of the fat-soluble vitamins (the other fat-soluble ones are D, E and K). It occurs naturally in fish liver oils. Most of the vitamin A in use today is synthetically produced, the form used largely in vitamin preparations as well as in the enrichment of foods, as milk powder, margarine and animal feeds. It is by virtue of its tastelessness that the synthetic vitamin A can be used in food enrichment. Can you imagine how few people would use enriched foods if the vitamin A enrichment was from cod liver oil?

As with other synthetic vitamins there is no difference in effect between them and the naturally derived vitamins. Either will protect against deficiency and either will overcome symptoms of deficiency when they occur. (An exception will be discussed under vitamins B.)

Vitamin A is stored in the liver in the form of an ester—a chemical combination of an acid and an alcohol. It is more stable in that form than in the pure form and is drawn from the body as needed. The liver thus acts as a sort of bank or depository. It is also stored in other tissues of the body.

Since vitamin A is a fat-soluble vitamin it needs two substances for its absorption: fat, to mix with it (from which mixture it is absorbed by the tissues), and bile acids, which come from the gallbladder and emulsify fats to make them utilizable by absorption.

Vitamin A is easily destroyed by oxidation—i.e., when it is exposed to the air for an appreciable period of time. That is the reason why cod liver oil, a rich source of natural vitamin A, was usually kept under refrigeration after the bottle was opened. It did not need the cold but it did need a tightly closed bottle to exclude air. But the cold did help some in delaying the oxi-

dation of the oil. For that reason many of the preparations of
vitamin A used today—cod liver oil is hardly used now as a supplementary source of vitamin A—contain antioxidants, such as
vitamin E, lecithin or BHT (butylated hydroxytoluene). They
retard the oxidation of vitamin A. Today's preparations, which
are usually in the form of capsules, do not need special storage
as they are not exposed to air and, in addition, are protected
against oxidation by the minute quantities of these antioxidants.

In What Foods Is Vitamin A Found?

Under ordinary circumstances your food should supply the
vitamin A you need to prevent deficiency. The sources are commonly available foods, at least in the affluent countries. But
apparently, as noted earlier, deficiencies do occur, probably because people do not choose an ideal diet.

And even if you do consume an ideal diet, some events such as
malabsorption may militate against your getting enough vitamin A. A balanced multivitamin preparation assures your receiving enough of the vitamins to prevent deficiency, even a sub-
clinical deficiency.

Do familiarize yourself with what foods contain what vitamins.
The advantages are obvious.

Vitamin A, being a fat-soluble vitamin, will be found in food
substances that contain fat. But there is an exception to that
point: carotene, which is a precursor to vitamin A, is found in
plants.

The strength of vitamin A is expressed in terms of international
units, usually written as IU. The amount that is necessary daily to
prevent deficiency differs (see inside front cover for RDA chart).

Bear in mind that there are substantial differences in vitamin content of foods due to seasons of the year. For example, butter or milk may contain twice as much vitamin A in summer as in winter. The amount of vitamin A listed below is rounded off because it would be a case of misplaced and pointless precision to state, for example, that kale, a rich source of vitamin A, contains 8,100 IU per cup, when the amount in a cup depends on how densely it is packed, how large the leaves, etc. Moreover, it is easier to remember 8,000, rather than to be in doubt if the figure you're trying to recall is 8,100 or 1,800. Cooking reduces the vitamin A potential in green vegetables about 20 percent and yellow vegetables about 30 percent.

Vitamin A Values

The following foods are rich in vitamin A: milk, egg yolk, liver, kidney, heart, butter, sea food, fish (especially fish livers), fortified margarine.

The following foods are rich in carotene: carrots, spinach, broccoli, escarole, cabbage, lettuce, kale, brussels sprouts, tomatoes.

The following listing of certain selected vitamin A-rich foods states the amount of vitamin A contained in the stated portion.

Due to fluctuation of vitamin A content of foods, dietary eccentricities or ethnic tastes, and more particularly in the light of the Ten-State Nutrition Survey, supplementation of the vitamin A intake would appear to be a wise step. Such supplementation is usually attained by the customary multivitamin capsules which contain, per capsule, from 5,000 IU to not more than 10,000 IU of vitamin A.

A recent regulation of the FDA cuts the amount of vitamin A sold over-the-counter without prescription to 10,000 IU vitamin A

		IU
milk: whole, 3.5% fat	1 cup	350
skim (not enriched)	1 cup	10
buttermilk, fluid, cultured, made from skim milk	1 cup	10
camembert cheese	1 wedge	380
cheddar cheese	1 oz	370
cottage cheese: creamed	4 oz	200
uncreamed	4 oz	10
cream cheese	3 oz	1,300
cream: half-and-half	1 cup	1,160
light	1 cup	2,000
sour	1 cup	1,930
for whipping, light	1 tbsp	190
for whipping, heavy	1 tbsp	230
yogurt: from whole milk	1 tbsp	340
from partly skimmed	1 tbsp	170
egg: 1 whole		580
1 yolk		580
beef, pot roasted (lean & fat)	3 oz	30
steak (sirloin), broiled, lean & fat	3 oz	50
steak (round), lean only	3 oz	20
liver, beef, fried	2 oz	30,280
swordfish, broiled with butter	3 oz	1,750
asparagus, cooked, drained	4 stalks	540
beet greens, leaves & stems, cooked & drained	1 cup	7,400
broccoli, cooked & drained	1 stalk	4,500
brussels sprouts	1 cup	800
carrots, grated	1 cup	12,000
collards, cooked	1 cup	10,250
dandelion greens, cooked	1 cup	21,000
kale, leaves & stalks, cooked	1 cup	8,000
spinach, cooked	1 cup	14,500
sweet potatoes, baked (approx. 6 oz.)	1 cup	9,000
butter or margarine	1 tbsp	470
	1 pat	170

per capsule. Compare this with liver—not under prescription strictures: only 2 ounces of fried beef liver contains about 30,000 IU vitamin A.

BRIEF POINTS ON VITAMIN A

Is deficiency frequent?	Yes
U.S. RDA per day	5,000 IU
Danger of overdose?	Infrequent but possible

6

THE NERVE VITAMINS—
THE VITAMINS B

WHILE THE VITAMINS B are loosely referred to as the *nerve vitamins* their deficiency is expressed in several systems of the body. For example, skin and hair disorders occur when there is a deficiency of most of the B vitamins. More particularly, skin changes occur in deficiencies of pantothenic acid, niacin, pyridoxine (B_6) and riboflavin (B_2). But more specific symptoms are associated with each vitamin as will be outlined.

Changes in the mouth, eye, reproductive glands, or anomalies of the utilization of other nutrients occur when there is either a deficiency of a given B vitamin or, through another process, an increased need. One such process is stress, which increases the need for the water-soluble B vitamins.

What we know of the results of deficiency of any of the B vitamins was first learned through experimentation on rats: these test animals were fed an otherwise fully adequate diet which was lacking only in a specific vitamin, and the resulting deficiency was noted. This knowledge was applied to man. But it does not mean that a specific observation of a deficiency in a rat or other animal always applies to man. For example, when a rat's fur becomes scraggly and hair begins to fall when deprived of pantothenic acid, it does not follow that an analogous skin condition in man is due to pantothenic acid deficiency. It may or may not be. Only specific observations in man apply to man, as another factor may be present. Even if a skin lesion is observed in man and is considerably improved by administration of pantothenic acid, it does not necessarily follow that there was a pantothenic acid deficiency. The improvement may have been due to the pharmacological effect of that vitamin and not due to a repair of a deficiency.

There are many components of the vitamin B complex, each of them being a vitamin B. They are distinguished by small inferior numerals after the B (as B_1, B_2, etc.) or in many instances by name (as nicotinic acid or niacin). These, then, are the components of the vitamin B complex as we know them today:

Vitamin B_1 or thiamine	Niacin or nicotinic acid
Vitamin B_2 or riboflavin	Folic acid
Vitamin B_6 or the pyridoxine group	Pantothenic acid
Vitamin B_{12} or the cobalamin group	Biotin

Questions may well be asked: What happened to the numbers between vitamins B_1 and B_{12}? Who is hoarding them? And didn't I hear once of a vitamin B_{15}? You did.

In the early history of vitamin development consecutive numbers were assigned to each new discovery of one of the B vitamins. Thus, for example, references exist to the nutritional values of vitamins B_3, B_4, B_5, B_7, B_8, B_{10}, B_{12}, B_{13}, B_{14}, B_{15}. Many of these factors were found to be nutritionally useful in rats, chickens or pigeons. Vitamin B_3 was believed to be pantothenic acid, then nicotinic acid; in fact B_5 was found to be probably identical with nicotinic acid. Similarly, vitamin P is no longer considered to be a vitamin. Another example: vitamin M or vitamin Bc and vitamin U are obsolete names for folic acid or folacin.

Subsequently, a number of growth factors were identified which were found eventually to be similar to or identical with an already known vitamin; for example, a substance first named vitamin Y turned out to be identical with the already known vitamin B_6, or pyridoxine. Similarly, vitamin G is now solely called vitamin B_2 or riboflavin.

Other substances, used today and found essential, have been given more descriptive names. For example, the essential fatty acids which are not vitamins, such as linolenic and linoleic acids, were once designated vitamin F, and in some parts of the world are still referred to by that name. There are other substances found in the vitamin B complex such as choline or inositol. They do perform certain vitaminlike functions in metabolism but are not considered vitamins. All of the B vitamins are water-soluble, including even riboflavin which, though extremely difficult to dissolve in water, dissolves when nicotinic acid is added.

VITAMIN B_1, OR THIAMINE

While the classical deficiency sign of B_1, namely beriberi, is not found in the United States, other signs of a low utilization or low intake of B_1 do occur.

The reason for deficiency may be obviously low intake of B_1, or the intake may be too low because the carbohydrate intake is too high. The more carbohydrate that is taken, the greater the need for B_1. Certain conditions, such as high thyroid activity, may increase the need for additional B_1. One of the outstanding reasons for thiamine deficiency or malutilization is alcoholism.

Thiamine deprivation due to high alcoholic intake affects the function of nerves and muscle tissue. The arm pain of alcoholics is well known. Many develop heart dysfunction which rapidly progresses. Mental confusion frequently develops when alcoholism, even though not severe, has long continued. Muscle cramps or weakness, numbness and eventually paralysis may occur due to thiamine deprivation. But thiamine does not cure the sequels of alcoholism. In alcoholism there is also a deficiency of other water-soluble B vitamins as B_2, B_6, folic acid, as well as certain minerals or micronutrients, particularly magnesium, potassium and zinc. However, Wernicke's syndrome and peripheral neuritis do respond to B_1.

Thiamine may also be involved in other disease conditions. For example, the severity of diabetes is increased on a low thiamine intake. As a matter of fact, thiamine deficiency may be implicated in eye dysfunction in nondiabetic as well as diabetic individuals. In thiamine deficiency a neuritis of the eye (retrobulbar neuritis) may occur as well as paralysis of the muscles of the eye which are responsible for the mobility of the eyeball.

It appears, too, that thiamine in association with other B vitamins actually aids in overcoming the night blindness in vitamin A deficiency. There are reports that vitamin A, the so-called eye vitamin, has not been effective alone in relieving night blindness, but together with the administration of the B vitamins rapidly increases the ability to see in semidarkness. Other common signs of thiamine deficiency are lack of appetite, weight loss and fatigue, though these symptoms may also be due to other causes.

How Does Deficiency Arise?

Deficiency may arise through low intake of the vitamin, high intake of calories, particularly carbohydrates, and as a result of certain other conditions such as overactivity of the thyroid and stress. Stress—including surgery, exposure to cold or other conditions—increases the need for water-soluble vitamins, especially the B vitamins. Other periods of stress are adolescence, aging and pregnancy.

A low vitamin level can also arise when the level of enzyme that converts it (transketolase) is low, or if the body poorly utilizes the enzyme that aids in its conversion. There may even be an adequate level of thiamine in blood yet its utilization may be insufficient as one of the enzymes helping its utilization is not active. Another reason for inadequate utilization of thiamine may be lack of or, more likely, an insufficient amount of magnesium, one of the minerals that aid in the activity of the converting enzymes.

But have in mind that neither thiamine nor any other *single* vitamin deficiency may be involved. In these malutilizations—as in alcoholism, for example—deficiencies of several of the B vitamins exist at one time.

What Does Thiamine Do?

Thiamine is principally involved in energy metabolism. To that end, in concert with the enzymes that aid in its conversion, it facilitates the utilization of starches and sugars, i.e., carbohydrates, converting them into energy and fat. This does not mean that B_1 is "fattening." Fat is necessary in the common daily metabolic interchanges that takes place. It is not the B_1 that is fattening but the excess of carbohydrate intake.

Increased requirements may be necessary under conditions such as work at high temperature, which produces sweating. Many water-soluble substances are lost in sweat—including certain minerals, micronutrients as well as vitamins—so it would be wise to increase the thiamine intake under those conditions.

A grave occasion of stress is when one is undergoing surgery.

At that time the total nutritional picture must be assessed for many nutrients. Proteins and increased carbohydrates are particularly necessary before and after surgery. But an increased carbohydrate intake requires more thiamine; so if glucose or dextrose is administered intravenously, a combination of water-soluble B vitamins is usually given in the intravenous solution.

The B vitamins, being water-soluble, are not found in fats such as butter but in food having a high proportion of water.

The strength of B_1, as with all B vitamins except one, is expressed in milligrams (mg) and fractions of a milligram. The only exception is B_{12}, which is expressed in micrograms (mcg). A microgram is 1/1000 of a milligram or a millionth of a gram. There are 28,000 milligrams to an ounce, making a gram about 1/28 of an ounce and a milligram about 1/28,000 of an ounce.

For Recommended Daily Allowances (RDA) of the B vitamins, see inside front cover.

Vitamin B_1 Values

The following foods are rich in vitamin B_1: yeast, enriched or whole grain products or whole cereals, liver, lean pork, and fresh green vegetables. But overcooking reduces or may even destroy it. Milk is a fairly good source but human milk is poor. Nonenriched flour, cereals and white rice are poor in or devoid of B_1 content.

BRIEF POINTS ON VITAMIN B_1

Is deficiency frequent?	Not often
U.S. RDA?	1.5 mg
Danger of overdose?	Rare

The following listing of certain selected foods rich in the vitamins B states the amounts of thiamine (B_1), riboflavin (B_2) and niacin contained in the stated portions:

		MILLIGRAMS (MG)		
		B_1	B_2	Niacin
Milk, whole, 3.5% fat	1 cup	0.07	0.44	0.2
Milk, skim	1 cup	0.09	0.44	0.2
Yeast, dry, baker's active	7 gm pkg	0.16	0.38	2.6
Yeast, dry, brewer's	8 gm tbsp	1.25	0.34	3.0
Beef, pot roast, lean & fat	3 oz	0.04	0.18	3.5
Steak, broiled, sirloin, lean & fat	3 oz	0.05	0.16	4.0
Steak, broiled, round, lean only	3 oz	0.08	0.20	5.0
Liver, beef, fried	2 oz	0.15	2.35	9.4
Swordfish, broiled with butter	3 oz	0.03	0.04	9.3
Egg	1	0.05	0.15	—
Barley, pearled, light, uncooked	200 gm	0.24	0.10	6.2
Bread: white, soft crumb type	1 slice	0.06	0.05	0.6
white, firm crumb type	1 slice	0.06	0.05	0.6
whole wheat, soft crumb type	1 slice	0.09	0.03	0.8
whole wheat, firm crumb type	1 slice	0.06	0.03	0.7
Oatmeal or rolled oats, cooked	240 gm	0.19	0.05	0.2
Broccoli, whole medium stalks	1 stalk	0.16	0.36	1.4
Brussels sprouts	1 cup	0.12	0.22	1.2
Orange juice, fresh	1 cup	0.22	0.07	1.0
Cornmeal, whole-ground unbolted, dry	1 cup	0.46	0.13	2.4

VITAMIN B_2, OR RIBOFLAVIN

Deficiency of B_2 is commonly thought of as pellagra, but it produces other complaints. Some of these are expressed as malfunction of the eyes (e.g., intolerance to light and "road-maps" on the cornea), eyes that show many red streaks and itching or burning. Other signs are skin changes, particularly lesions in the corner of the mouth called cheilosis, inflammation of the tongue called glossitis, and anemia. Many of these are similar to the changes also brought about by niacin deficiency, and it is difficult to determine if a deficiency is due to B_2 alone or to a combination deficiency with other B vitamins.

Vitamin B_2 deficiency can be characterized by dysfunction in three large areas: physiological stress, resistance and infection. An outstanding characteristic of B_2 deficiency may well be the occurrence of birth defects. This has clearly been determined in animals. That the same relationship applies to human beings is not clear, but quite probably it does. (See Chapter 15, "Pigs Without Eyeballs: Birth Defects.")

Unlike B_1, there is no increased need for B_2 when the caloric intake increases. But there is a similar relationship with protein intake—B_2 is necessary for the building of tissue, which proteins serve. It is also necessary to guard against infections, such as those that are produced by deficiency of B_2—as lesions on corners of the mouth (cheilosis). Diabetics whose disease is not controlled often suffer a B_2 deficiency. In other words, lesions of deficiency appear in the mouth, eye and skin. Another characteristic sign of B_2 deficiency is skin lesions of the scrotum. However, such signs may indicate other conditions. For example, lesions of the corners of the mouth may also be due to ill-fitting dentures. Neither B_2 nor any other vitamin will remedy that.

Alcoholics hit the bottle and B vitamin deprivation hits the alcoholic. The alcoholic is deprived of all water-soluble B vitamins as a result of reduced food intake (in the case of B_1 there is, in addition, an increased need to metabolize alcohol). Thus the need of the alcoholic is not for B_2 alone, but for all the B vitamins.

What Does B_2 Do?

That riboflavin is "good for the eyes" is true, but it is an over-simplification. More broadly, riboflavin, as well as niacin, is considered an *electron-transfer vitamin*, in that it is needed for the biochemical events in the body that enable the liberation of energy for cell function to take place. In addition, riboflavin is also involved in the utilization of foodstuffs, most likely in the metabolism of fatty acids, which are also involved in energy metabolism.

As with other water-soluble B vitamins, B_2 is found in milk and other dairy foods, enriched or whole grain products or cereals, liver, lean meat, fresh green vegetables, eggs. (See list under vitamin B_1 for food values.)

BRIEF POINTS ON VITAMIN B_2

Is deficiency frequent?   No
U.S. RDA?   1.7 mg
Danger of overdose?   Rare

NIACIN, OR NICOTINIC ACID

Niacin is the antipellagra vitamin—and then some. It is far-reaching in its double-barreled effect both in the multiplicity and severity of signs of deficiency and in its pharmacological action.

Pellagra is a disease of corn-eating regions and is presumably now rarely found in the United States, but in other parts of the world it is not rare. Attacking three systems, it is characterized by the three D's—dermatitis (skin), diarrhea (gastrointestinal) and dementia (nervous system). Its deficiency often shows milder symptoms. For example, there are changes in the mouth in the event of deficiency—inflammation and other changes in the mucous membrane, including inflammation of the tongue (glossitis). Skin changes can occur on any part of the body, appearing as hard, dry, scaly skin or as brown pigmentation, redness or even swelling.

Though pellagra as a nutritional disease in the United States, particularly the corn-eating South, has been wiped out as an epidemic with its classical DDD signs, it probably does occur mildly in different forms. It is not the result of corn eating, but we must return to alcoholism, which strips the individual of his much-needed B vitamins, producing a special kind, alcoholic pellagra. Also, the compulsion to reduce body weight on the part of the adolescent girl often leads her to bizarre diets with impending malnutrition, including B_2 deficiency. In these instances, deficiency may appear as weakness, abdominal pains, headache, irritability and sleeplessness or even a red and furry tongue, and mentally "not-being-with-it."

What Does Niacin Do?

Note that there are *niacin,* also called nicotinic acid, and *niacinamide,* also called nicotinic acid amide or nicotinamide. To prevent nutritional deficiency, either is equally suitable and serves the same purpose. (For reducing the cholesterol level or for increasing peripheral circulation in the aging, niacin only is used.) For food enrichment, niacinamide is commonly used.

Tryptophan, an amino acid, occurs in foods and can give niacin an identity problem. It can actually be curative in pellagra because tryptophan converts to niacin by a system of intricate biochemical steps. But it is not practical: tryptophan is extremely high in price and is not efficient to use in place of niacin, because it takes 60 parts tryptophan to make 1 part of niacin.

Similar to riboflavin, nictinic acid is also an *electron-transfer vitamin,* acting as an energizer to make the enzymes needed for oxidation-reduction reactions, carbohydrate metabolism, other energy conversion, and for tryptophan metabolism which has other tasks to perform in addition to conversion to niacin. It is a complex cycle, and if pellagra does not make you dizzy, this complexity will.

Thus niacin is vital in the normal function of the central nervous system, in guarding the integrity of the skin and mucous membrane, and more particularly in supplying the needed coenzyme for the energy cycles.

Foods

One cannot consider what foods contain niacin without recognizing the role of tryptophan. For that reason, niacin in foods is expressed as *niacin equivalents*. Part of the total of the niacin is due to niacin or niacinamide and part to tryptophan—1/60 of which is a *niacin equivalent*. For example, cow's milk contains 12 mg niacin equivalents per 1,000 calories, of which 1.2 mg is due to niacin and the remainder to tryptophan. This is another reason why food as a totality rather than a vitamin per se should be the aim of good nutrition.

Niacin is much more stable to heat and light than B_1 or B_2.

Foods

Niacin is found in milk and other dairy products, eggs, lean beef, liver, whole grain cereals (especially those enriched with niacin), yeast, fish, as tuna and salmon, lima beans, peanuts. (See list under vitamin B_1 for food values.)

You may have heard of niacin or niacinamide referred to as vitamin B_3 for the treatment of schizophrenia. This was originated by Drs. Humphry Osmond and Abram Hoffer, who continue to report outstanding success with it. Several other investigators reported that they cannot duplicate the results claimed by Osmond and Hoffer.

New ideas commonly find detractors. In such a puzzling and grave condition as schizophrenia, where there is little curative that can be offered, serious and concerted attention should be broadly given to niacin therapy. By sheer numbers and long follow-up, niacin should eventually either be found to be one of the best answers we now have or be completely rejected for that purpose. Instead, there continue to be differences of opinion and wrangling. The enemy is schizophrenia, not a competing investigator.

Osmond and Hoffer consider schizophrenia a biochemical anomaly. Other investigators have different views as to its cause: genetic, psychogenic, environmental, etc. It is entirely possible that schizophrenia is actually a group of diseases having different facets. One or more such variants may be responsive to treatment by niacin.

BRIEF POINTS ON NIACIN

U.S. RDA?	20 mg
Danger of overdose?	Rare

VITAMIN B$_6$, OR PYRIDOXINE

Vitamins generally are looked upon as protection against deficiency. Some, however, have a pharmacological action beyond that, i.e., they have a therapeutic effect of their own. One such vitamin is B$_6$.

In a comparatively rare condition which is in the group of disorders called errors of metabolism, B$_6$ is literally a lifesaver. When this condition is found in infants, comparatively large daily quantities of vitamin B$_6$ overcome the error of metabolism, which could produce convulsions leading to brain damage and resulting in death.

A metabolic error (or inborn error of metabolism) is a genetic condition in which nature slipped a cog and did not provide for a certain enzyme needed for the orderly events in metabolism to take place. Such an enzyme is missing—and therefore cannot enter the normal metabolic reactions.

While the picture of B$_6$ deficiency is not as dramatic as that of other B vitamins, it nonetheless exists, though it occurs infrequently in the United States. Among B$_6$ deficiency symptoms, which also may be due to other causes, are dysfunctions of the skin or nervous system and infection. The skin symptoms of B$_6$ deficiency are eczemalike outbreaks which may occur on the face and ears or anywhere on the body. Some of them resemble the skin symptoms found in deficiency of niacin, but are not cured by niacin. The nervous symptoms include fatigue and lethargy, and neuritis which results when certain drugs are given which act as B$_6$ antagonists. A type of conjunctivitis and inflammation of the eyelids is precipitated by B$_6$ deficiency, which clears up when B$_6$ is taken. Mental retardation in children and dulling of memory in adults have been described as sequels of B$_6$ deficiency.

Its deficiency in animals has wider ramifications in that the symptoms affect other body systems as well (such as muscles). For example, in rats pregnancy cannot continue when there is B_6 deficiency. Growth is also inhibited, and other animals, like dogs, develop a type of anemia which responds only to B_6.

What Does B_6 Do?

Vitamin B_6 may in fact be more broadly involved in the body economy than its deficiency symptoms suggest. It is necessary in the enzymatic function of the cell, as, for example, in the body synthesis of DNA, one of the life nucleic acids; it is necessary in amino acid metabolism, hence in protein and also fat metabolism, as well as that of certain hormones.

Together with another member of the B complex group, namely, pantothenic acid, deficiency of B_6 reduces immunity to attack by diphtheria or other organisms which depends upon immunological protection. While this effect was primarily observed in animals, it is believed by some, though not by others, that B_6 is involved in the protection that immunity confers. The reason for this reduction of immunity may be because its deficiency impairs DNA and RNA synthesis.

Infants at times develop convulsions not related to the inborn errors of metabolism previously mentioned, but as a result of depletion of B_6 in the feeding formula. One such event in epidemic proportions took place in the 1950's in which a formula for infant feeding was B_6 deficient due to processing. Infants recover quickly when B_6 is added to their diet.

In alcoholics there is a marked deficiency in all of the B vitamins but B_6 has a special place: the convulsions that often occur in sudden alcohol withdrawal may be due to irritability of the nervous system which accompanies alcoholism. In addition, B_6

(together with B_1) is also needed for the oxidation process to metabolize alcohol.

There are other conditions in which B_6 has been often used with success. Vomiting in pregnancy has long been treated with large doses. B_6 has been described as necessary to many of the functions of the brain, which is not surprising when we remember its relation to convulsions. The following need extra B_6 for optimum function: women taking oral contraceptives, who also need extra vitamin C, B_{12} and folic acid; those taking antidepressants or isoniazid (a drug used in the treatment of tuberculosis); and those with certain anemias.

The intake of given nutrients often affects the need of certain vitamins and may increase the requirements. The need of B_1 is increased with an increased intake of carbohydrate. A similar situation occurs with B_6: the higher the intake of protein, the greater the need of B_6. The reason is based upon the presence of two amino acids: the more methionine or tryptophan, both necessary amino acids found in protein, the greater the amount of B_6 needed.

Vitamin B_6 is an aggregate name for three substances: pyridoxine (which is the name usually on the label of multivitamin preparations), pyridoxal and pyridoxamine. All have the activity of B_6.

Foods

The following foods are rich in B_6: beef liver, kidney, pork loin and ham, leg of veal, fresh fish, bananas, cabbage, avocados, peanuts, walnuts, raisins and prunes, wheat germ (very rich), soybean flour, brown rice, split peas. Milk and eggs contain only fair amounts.

(See Recommended Daily Allowance of B_6 on inside front cover.)

BRIEF POINTS ON VITAMIN B_6

U.S. RDA?	2 mg
Danger of overdose?	No

PANTOTHENIC ACID

The name itself, pantothenic acid, implies the wide distribution of the vitamin (*pan*—all, everywhere). While deficiency symptoms in rats, mice, chickens and other animals are well known, it was difficult to produce pantothenic acid deficiency in man until the middle 1950's. Then it was produced by feeding an antivitamin or vitamin antagonist, namely, omega-methylpantothenic acid (see antivitamins, in Chapter 18), which antagonizes the effects of pantothenic acid and produces a deficiency.

The symptoms of such deficiency in man are fatigue and lethargy, headache, general malaise, sleep disturbance, nausea, vomiting and abdominal discomfort. In alcoholics, who are particularly susceptible to deficiency of B vitamins, the symptoms probably include nerve disturbances such as reduced sensation in arms or legs. Often it is difficult to determine whether a deficiency is that of B_6 or pantothenic acid.

In animals, the signs of deficiency are skin and nervous system abnormalities. The adrenal glands undergo destructive changes in case of deficiency. In view of the close relationship between the adrenals and stress, it is deduced that pantothenic acid is especially necessary in the protection from stress—similar to vitamin C. Other damages in various animals from pantothenic acid deficiency are incoordination, muscle spasm, and brain inflammation. In a famous experiment with black rats, their hair turned gray but was restored to its former glistening black by administration of the vitamin. Based on that observation, people took pantothenic acid to restore gray hair to its former color—with disappointing results. Animals with pantothenic acid deficiency have a low level of coenzyme A in their tissues—one of the irreplaceable enzymes in the body economy.

As with other B vitamins, the need for pantothenic acid in the treatment of alcoholics is imperative.

What Does Pantothenic Acid Do?

Its considerable value for man lies in its role in the enzyme system of the body as it is part of coenzyme A, a most important enzyme which is related to the utilization of nutrients, hence production of energy. Pantothenic acid is also involved in the integrity of the nervous system and the function of the gastrointestinal tract. Another of its functions is its role in human immunity, protecting the system against attack by bacterial invaders. The body produces antibodies against certain toxins; deficiency of pantothenic acid (as well as other vitamins) inhibits this ability. While much more of this activity is known in animals, much applies to man. For example, pantothenic acid deficiency reduces production of antibodies to tetanus antigen (toxin). This inhibition becomes worse if there is a multiple deficiency, i.e., of both pantothenic acid and B_6.

Pantothenic acid has been more recently reported to be useful to promote well-being in other conditions. For example, in pregnancy, especially in teenagers, it is particularly desirable as its blood level was found higher in nonpregnant teenagers than in pregnant ones. (See also Chapter 15 on birth defects.)

Because of its role in the function of the adrenals, it is a persuasive argument that an adequate amount of pantothenic acid together with vitamin A can aid in preventing the damage that stress can produce. The adrenals are directly involved in stress and can be depleted in long-continued stress.

Foods

The following foods are rich in pantothenic acid: beef, lamb, pork liver, kidney, broccoli, kale, avocados, split peas, lentils, lima beans, cashew nuts, walnuts, egg yolk, yeast, wheat bran, and oats. Milk contains only fair amounts.

BRIEF POINTS ON PANTOTHENIC ACID

U.S. RDA?	10 mg
Danger of overdose?	Rare

BIOTIN

Occasionally referred to by the unacceptable name of vitamin H, biotin is widely distributed in nature, and as with pantothenic acid, deficiency signs had to be induced in order to observe what they were.

In man, the deficiency induced by feeding egg whites or foods low in biotin produced symptoms similar to pantothenic acid deficiency: lethargy, sleepiness, muscle pain and numbness of some parts of the body, eczemalike skin outbreaks, paleness of skin and mucous membrane, then gastrointestinal symptoms, such as loss of appetite and nausea.

In animals the same symptoms are more severe, in addition to which there are loss of hair and reduction of growth, hardening of the eyelids, learning inhibition, spasm and partial paralysis of hind legs. These were produced by feeding almost solely raw egg whites. For that reason one of the early names for biotin was *egg white injury factor*. This is not due to the poisonous nature of egg white but to one of its ingredients, avidin, which acts as an interfering factor in the synthesis of biotin in the intestine.

Foods

Biotin is produced in the intestine of man and other animals and, like pantothenic acid, is widely distributed in nature. It is most plentiful in liver, kidney, egg yolks and many fresh vegetables.

BRIEF POINTS ON BIOTIN

U.S. RDA?	0.3 mg
Danger of overdose?	Rare

FOLIC ACID

The terms *folic acid* and *folacin* refer to the same substance. Another name, though not frequently used, is PGA (pteroylglutamic acid), which is chemically descriptive. Folinic acid (also called citrovorum factor or leucovorin) is a variant with the effect of folic acid. The term *folate* can mean any of the preceding.

Deficiency can produce a type of anemia in both man and other animals. Since it is a vitamin (similar to B_6 and B_{12}) that is directly related to the synthesis of DNA and other nucleic acids, its other deficiency symptoms are equally broad and rapidly develop when there is deficiency of or inadequate folacin in the diet: in addition to anemia, neuritis occurs in folacin deficiency in adults, and behavioral difficulties, irritability, even convulsions in infants. Another result of deficiency may be inadequate brain development with neurological deficit. Birth defects are among the grave results of deficiency in pregnant women. (See Chapter 15 on birth defects.)

There is general agreement among authorities that all pregnant women should receive supplemental folacin. Pregnant women taking other drugs need more folacin according to Russell K. Laros, Jr., M.D., of the University of Michigan.

Many oral contraceptives produce a deficiency of folacin and anemia, according to the Council on Foods and Nutrition of the American Medical Association. Hence, women who are taking oral contraceptives should receive folacin supplements. Most knowledgeable people agree that such women should also take other vitamins such as vitamins C, B_6, B_{12}.

Deficiency of folacin as well as of B_{12} and B_6 can produce stomach irritation, inflammation of the tongue and inhibition of wound healing by retarding the formation of the vitally basic nucleic acids, DNA and RNA.

What Does Folacin or Folate Do?

Folacin matures red blood cells, preventing certain anemias— in fact, several types of anemia. The anemia of alcoholics must be treated with folacin, but the need of other B vitamins is not thereby reduced. Provided that the intake of alcohol is discontinued, the anemia can be reversed.

Folacin prevents and treats three different kinds of anemia. I hope no one uses this as a headline because these anemias are not for self-treatment (nutritional macrocytic, macrocytic anemia of pregnancy, and in infants, megaloblastic anemia). Folate was at one time used in the treatment of the dread pernicious anemia; while it treated the anemia adequately, it allowed the neurological degeneration to continue. Therefore, B_{12} is now used in pernicious anemia, with or without folacin.

Thus folacin prevents the fatigue and loss of appetite, shortness of breath, swelling of the membranes of the mouth that accompany these folate-responding anemias. It also has a role in the metabolism of proteins.

Immunity to certain infectious diseases is dependent on many factors. In common with pantothenic acid and B_6, folate prevents the impairment of immunological defenses of the body.

In pregnancy there is an increased need for folic acid (among other vitamins). The fetus drains the pregnant mother of much of her folacin stores, so she needs supplementation daily. It is estimated that half the pregnant women in the world may be folacin deficient.

Other drugs can interfere with folate utilization. Such drugs as isoniazid for tuberculosis, methotrexate for certain forms of cancer, or diphenylhydantoin for epilepsy can call forth folate deficiency. Another condition that responds is tropical sprue, a disease originating in the tropics but found elsewhere in the world as well. It is characterized by swollen tongue, digestive and other gastrointestinal dysfunctions. (Folate, folacin and folic acid are terms that may be used interchangeably.)

Foods

Folic acid—so named because it was originally found in green leaves (*folia*—leaves)—is widely dispersed in nature. While there is rarely a deficiency with other widely available vitamins such as pantothenic acid and biotin, that is not true of folate. One reason for the widespread deficiency, especially in pregnant women or those taking oral contraceptives, is the increased need for folate under those conditions.

Folate occurs plentifully, especially in liver and kidney, round steak, wheat germ and other wheat products as wheat bran or shredded wheat, yeast, green leafy vegetables as spinach, broccoli, endive, Swiss chard, asparagus, black-eyed peas, lima and red kidney beans and particularly in orange juice. Destroyed by high heat or long cooking, folate is best retained under refrigeration while the food is awaiting preparation.

(See RDA for folacin on inside front cover.)

BRIEF POINTS ON FOLACIN

Deficiency frequent?	Yes
U.S. RDA?	0.4 mg
Danger of overdose?	Rare, but in pernicious anemia if given without B_{12} allows neurological damage to proceed.

VITAMIN B_{12}, OR COBALAMINS

Vitamin B_{12} is called the pernicious anemia vitamin but it has other functions as well. The terms *cyanocobalamin* and *hydroxocobalamin* both have the activity of B_{12}—they are B_{12}.

A deficiency of B_{12} leads to pernicious anemia. This may be due to lack of B_{12} in the diet or to a genetic factor in which intrinsic factor is lacking or deficient or a metabolic block exists in utilizing it.

Intrinsic factor is protein found in the stomach juice of man and in certain other animals such as swine—at least one link between the human and the porcine species. If there is no intrinsic factor present, pernicious anemia develops, as it is necessary for the absorption and utilization of B_{12}.

There are other symptoms of pernicious anemia besides the characteristic deformity of the red blood cells. One is degeneration of nerves, leading to neuritis, incoordination, and impairment of eye nerves, hence sight. Another is inflammation of the gastrointestinal tract including the stomach and the mucous membranes of the food pipe up into the mouth, as well as swelling of the mouth and tongue. Even mental confusion leading to psychosis may happen in pernicious anemia—the damage is widespread.

What Does B_{12} Do?

As with B_6 and folate, B_{12} is involved in the formation of nucleic acids, DNA and RNA, and important enzymes concerned with their functions. It is probably the most powerful nutrient—used in *microgram* quantities. Note how small: a microgram is $1/1000$ of a milligram, and a milligram is $1/1000$ of a gram—and there are 28.35 grams to an ounce.

After certain surgical procedures, as the removal of part of the stomach or of the small intestine, various digestive or other systemic dysfunctions may develop as the absorption of B_{12} is inhibited. These symptoms are ameliorated by giving B_{12}—which may be needed for the rest of the lives of these people. Other nutrients including vitamins and protein are also needed; because of removal of parts of the small intestine, malabsorption of many foods develops with diarrhea and fatty stools. Much larger doses of B_{12} are necessary in overcoming these conditions than in pernicious anemia.

While supplemental folate is necessary during pregnancy, this is usually not the case with B_{12}, though some pregnant women show an individual need for extra B_{12} during pregnancy.

Some investigators believe that in aging a greater amount of B_{12} is needed than in youth; others dispute this belief. But all agree that B_{12} stimulates appetite, weight and growth in children, especially when their general nutrition is not optimum.

Another condition that responds to B_{12} is fish-tapeworm anemia, as these tapeworms get to the B_{12} before the host.

The vegetarian fad has found an increasing number of adherents, based upon religious or "ethical" considerations or upon no other consideration except for peers adhering to a vegetarian diet. This may well produce B_{12} deficiency, since B_{12} is found only in animal products—meat, milk, cheese, eggs.

An increased need for B_{12} also occurs when oral contraceptives are taken—another example of the interrelationship of B_{12} with folate.

Foods

Vitamin B_{12} does not occur in vegetable matter, only in foods of animal sources. The richest source is liver. Another rich source is kidney, and round beef is good, though not as good a source as the organ meats. Shellfish, particularly oysters, are rich sources, as is camembert cheese; milk and eggs are satisfactory but not optimum sources. B_{12} is largely retained in cooking.

(See RDA for B_{12} on inside front cover.)

BRIEF POINTS ON VITAMIN B$_{12}$

Deficiency frequent?	No
U.S. RDA?	6 mcg.
Danger of overdose?	No

Natural vs. Synthetic

It was stated in the chapter on vitamin A that there is no difference in effect between vitamins derived from natural sources and those produced synthetically. Either will protect against deficiency and either will overcome symptoms of deficiency when they occur. There is one possible exception to this idea: a source such as yeast, which contains most B vitamins, may possibly contain an as yet unidentified B vitamin or an unknown factor that enhances the effect of the vitamins contained therein. This is not at all certain but conceivable.

This does not mean that, for example, thiamine derived from yeast is different from or preferable to that synthetically produced. It merely means that yeast or perhaps wheat germ, which is also rich in many B vitamins, may possibly contain a factor whose existence we do not suspect.

7

THE CELLULAR VITAMIN—VITAMIN C

IN COMMON with other vitamins, vitamin C collected several labels in its upward mobility to its current status. It started life as the antiscorbutic vitamin, and indeed it protects against scurvy and even cures if scurvy develops. Another name is the cellular vitamin, because it assures the wholeness of cells and tissues; for example, it protects against capillary breakage. But its functions are greater than the limits these two labels impose. Let us look into some of the other functions of vitamin C, which is also known as ascorbic acid.

Vitamin C is necessary for the following: wound healing, integrity of capillaries, growth and development of blood vessels, teeth, bones and other tissues. It is necessary in the development as well as the continuation of the all-important cell glue, the cement substance within the cell and between cells that holds cells together. Vitamin C is also irreplaceable in certain metabolic events since many reactions within the cell cannot proceed without it, though it needs other metabolites as well.

It is probably necessary for the healthy functioning of the adrenal gland, which together with the pituitary gland (the adrenal-pituitary axis) controls reproduction and smooth functioning of many gland-related activities. Vitamin C is probably vital in these organs, as they contain the highest concentration of vitamin C in the body. Other tissues in the body that contain a relatively high amount of vitamin C are eye, ovaries and testes, white blood cells, liver and brain. Apparently, it has inward as well as upward mobility.

Vitamin C—a natural, water-soluble antioxidant (vitamin E is a natural oil-soluble antioxidant)—is relatively nontoxic. As long ago as 1952 Lowry and his coworkers found that the intake of 1 gm (1,000 mg) per day by man, for months, had no bad effect. If the body has a sufficient supply, the rest is excreted. And it puts an arrowhead on iron: vitamin C increases the absorption and utilization of iron when given together with it.

Incidentally, in determining the vitamin C level in man it was found that the amount in the blood is not the same as that in the tissues, and physiologically it is the saturation in the tissues that counts. But its level can be best assessed in a component of the blood, namely, the platelets. Saturation can be assessed by excretion in the urine; if much is excreted it means the body has enough.

Methods of determination of vitamin C are used to verify that there is an adequate supply in the body. For example, after hemodialysis, i.e., "purifying" the blood by passing it through an artificial kidney, the vitamin C level is virtually depleted.

Serious things can happen in vitamin C deficiency, the most dreaded of which is scurvy. We probably have little or no obvious scurvy in the United States, but a mild form of scurvy is seen in hospitals, especially among the poor and the uneducated, or in infants, as well as the aged who live alone. The simple dietary cure is citrus fruit. The picture of scurvy has been historically recorded. Redness and sores on the skin developing into ulcers, swollen and bleeding gums and loss of teeth, bleeding into the skin, pain on moving, then inability just to move about because of profound weakness—this was the picture of sailors with scurvy. It is interesting to note that James Lind, a Scottish physician, described the treatment and cure of scurvy by lime juice in 1753, despite which it took the British Navy forty years more to dispense lime juice rations to its navy personnel. During this time large numbers of British sailors continued to die of scurvy.

Deficiency of vitamin C does not manifest itself as scurvy in the United States, but mild deficiencies do occur. Black-and-blue marks on the skin after a slight blow may be one expression of such mild deficiency.

What Does Vitamin C Do?

Aside from protecting against frank deficiency as exemplified by scurvy, vitamin C has additional functions. First, it is necessary in stress, in which there is an increased need for vitamin C. Pregnancy and lactation, inflammations and infections, burns, surgery, cold environment, high metabolic rate as in an overactive thyroid, diarrhea and considerably increased perspiration are among conditions in which there is an increased need for vitamin C, similar to the need for the water-soluble B vitamin in stress.

In wound healing from burns or from other causes different needs occur than in an otherwise normal state. There is an increased need for proteins, as well as for other vitamins and for certain ions such as sodium and potassium to prevent edema, which interferes with wound healing. Considerable vitamin C is also necessary in these conditions.

Old age is a stage in life when the organism does not cope with the stresses it has been able to handle during its prime. Hence, increased use in aging would seem to be logical.

It was pointed out by Hodges that emotional stress increases the need for vitamin C to double or triple the rate that individuals utilized under comparable situations but without emotional stress. This research was done in a prison, hence on a captive population in whom intake as well as utilization could be well controlled.

Other increased needs: The adrenal gland loses vitamin C upon stress. To maintain immunity and to facilitate the function of certain enzymes and vitamins—as, for example, to facilitate the function of folic acid—extra vitamin C is needed.

Alcoholics require many supports—nutritional, emotional and probably financial, as alcohol drains money as well as the water-soluble B vitamins. It also drains vitamin C, though not as crucially as it does the B vitamins. The need for extra vitamin C probably is caused by the high intake of alcohol, which has a high caloric value. Carbohydrates and proteins are equivalent to 4 calories per gram, but alcohol has 7 calories per gram, almost as much as fat, which is 9 calories per gram.

The infant, particularly the premature infant, requires an adequate intake of vitamin C, which is usually supplied in the diet, commonly by orange juice. At times infants are sensitive to orange juice, in which case vitamin C tablets serve admirably.

Every mammal can synthesize its own vitamin C except man, another dubious distinction he bears. His extra need is ever present. For example, the lens of the eye contains even more vitamin C than the adrenals and requires it for its healthy function. Even certain pustular infections of the aqueous component in the eye (aqueous humor) clear up by intake of vitamin C.

One of the few truly creative minds of our times is the distinguished Dr. Linus Pauling. Most of us are merely trained mechanics—whether it be in auto repair or in medicine—but truly inventive minds are rare. Pauling has proposed large doses of vitamin C in the prevention and treatment of colds, for which we have otherwise very little to offer. While many dissents from that view have been published, perhaps even more acclaim and successes have been experienced. It is our forecast that the use of vitamin C in the common cold will be accepted in the future. In some studies, such as the Anderson Toronto one, it seems already to have been vindicated.

The need for large quantities of vitamin C may in part be due to the differing needs of people. Dr. Roger J. Williams, a substantial figure in vitamin research, believes that owing to human variability, the needs are exponentially large for some people. In a lesser degree this may also apply to other animals. While monkeys and guinea pigs can synthesize vitamin C while man cannot produce vitamin C at all, they often cannot produce it fast enough to supply their own needs. Animals, other than monkeys and guinea pigs, can produce a sufficient amount for their own use.

Most interesting is the finding that vitamin C acts as an anticancer agent in bladder cancer. This was reported by a highly reputable urologist, Dr. J. U. Schlegel, working with a biochemist, Dr. George E. Pipkin, who found that 1.5 grams (1,500 mg) per day reverses the symptoms of bladder cancer. While this experience may possibly be eventually accepted, no confirmation or any other report has appeared since that first report in 1968.

Also unconfirmed, another important disease has been said to be amenable to treatment by vitamin C, namely, atherosclerosis. When it occurs in the arteries of the heart, it is called coronary atherosclerosis, in which there is deposition of cholesterol narrowing the blood vessels of the heart. A high amount of cholesterol is associated with an increased incidence of heart attacks. In the blood vessels of the brain the disease is called cerebral arteriosclerosis, which is hardening of the blood vessels (though it may also be atherosclerosis, which is deposition of cholesterol inside the blood vessels), and is characterized by partial loss of memory, confusion, and inappropriate behavior, leading to stroke.

Vitamin C has been recommended in doses of 1 gm (1,000 mg) daily to reduce the cholesterol level in the blood. One such study by the British Dr. Constance R. Spittle was done in man. Several other reports recount similar experiments in animals. But since other animals metabolize cholesterol differently from man, only work in human beings will actually settle the question.

While the use of vitamin C in the common cold has had a fair number of confirmations (the detractors had not used the large doses, i.e., 2 to 3 or more gm daily as originally prescribed by Dr. Pauling), vitamin C still appears wanting adequate confirmation in the reduction of cholesterol.

Its use in reducing the severity of the symptoms of allergy has been long reported. People with seasonal asthma increase their vitamin C intake at the time that their allergic symptoms recur. There are strong differences of opinion on the merits of vitamin C for allergy, but we wonder if both camps are speaking of the same thing: the reason for the doubt is that the proponents advocate huge doses of vitamin C, and the opponents regularly report little or no effect from the moderate doses they used in their studies.

Foods

The following foods are highly rich in vitamin C: citrus fruits, liver, spinach, tomatoes, most vegetables. You may not have known that fruits, except for citrus fruits, generally have a lower vitamin C content than vegetables.

Vitamin C is not destroyed by heat but by oxidation (heating with an access to air). Most of it is destroyed by holding prepared food on a steam table, as in ready-to-eat restaurants. Therefore, there is a substantial difference in the vitamin C content between raw and cooked vegetables.

Approximate Vitamin C Content of Selected Foods Expressed in Milligrams per 100 Grams of Food

Lemons	50
Oranges	50
Orange juice: fresh	140
frozen concentrate, undiluted	140
Limes	25
Liver	30
Mangos, raw	40
Guavas, raw	300
Kale: raw	110
cooked	50
Broccoli: raw	120
cooked	75
Brussels sprouts: raw	95
cooked	50
Potatoes: raw	20
cooked	15
boiled or baked	15
Cauliflower: raw	70
cooked	30
Grapefruit: raw	40
canned	30
Peppers, green: raw	120
cooked	100
Spinach: raw	60
cooked	30
Collards: raw	100
cooked	50
Turnip greens: raw	130
cooked	60
Asparagus: raw	35
cooked	20
Tomatoes: raw	25
canned	15

Compare with these low vitamin C foods per 100 grams of food:

Apple: raw	5 mg
cooked	1 mg
Lettuce	10 mg
Beets: raw	10 mg
cooked	5 mg

BRIEF POINTS ON VITAMIN C

Is deficiency frequent?	Mild form, yes
U.S. RDA?	60 mg
Danger of overdose?	No

The amount of a serving of a food makes a practical difference with respect to vitamin C intake. For example, parsley is very rich in vitamin C, containing 190 mg per 100 gm, or watercress 80 mg per 100 gm. But a serving of 3 oz of either is quite unrealistic. Note too that certain foods lend themselves to eating in the raw state, as cauliflower, which has about twice as much vitamin C raw as when cooked.

(See RDA for vitamin C on inside front cover.)

8

THE BONE VITAMIN—VITAMIN D

INDISPENSABLE FOR INFANTS and growing children, vitamin D is minimally necessary for adults. While it can be toxic in children in excessive doses, it can be even more toxic in adults who are taking even larger doses. Theoretically, one should be able to avoid the need for any supplementary vitamin D, because the body makes its own when exposed to sunlight. But the ultraviolet rays of sunlight which produce vitamin D are often blocked by weather or particulate matter in the atmosphere or reduced according to season of the year or altitude.

Vitamin D occurs naturally in fish liver oils. Cod liver oil was a standard item in the diet of infants and children not long ago. Today, vitamin D is a component of multivitamin preparations, and milk is fortified with 400 IU vitamin D per quart.

There are several effective forms of vitamin D. The most important and currently used are vitamin D_2 (irradiated ergosterol, calciferol) and vitamin D_3, which the body further converts to utilizable metabolites which have vitamin D activity. The effect of either type is about the same in human beings. In other animals one type differs from another. Since vitamin D is a fat-soluble vitamin, the intake of fat in the diet is necessary for its utilization.

Deficiency of vitamin D means rickets. The vitamin protects

against rickets but corrects its symptoms only if given early in infancy. Rickets is largely a disease of bone in infancy and childhood where the bones do not absorb calcium and phosphorus, with resulting malformations. The legs are bent, the head is somewhat misshapen, appearing square, the wrists are disproportionately enlarged, the abdomen as well as middle of chest (sternum) protrudes. The bowlegged adult had rickets as a child.

Vitamin D also is indispensable for the proper development of teeth and jawbone and the proper utilization of calcium and phosphorus—it is largely a bone vitamin. Both vitamin D and calcium are necessary to avoid rickets.

Rickets is not limited to its softening effect on bone. Another form of rickets affects the function of kidneys and the digestive apparatus, with spleen and liver enlargement—signs of malnutrition. This is known as vitamin D–resistant rickets, in which an immensely increased amount of vitamin D is necessary. The child having it is additionally loaded with a ponderous name, as it is also called *hypophosphatemic vitamin D–refractory rickets*. It is one of the metabolic errors whereby nature slipped a cog in the development of an enzyme system. Children with this type of rickets have a disturbance of calcium metabolism, as calcium does not deposit in bone.

Hence, rickets is a disease of deficiency of both vitamin D and calcium (vitamin D allows calcification to take place). Both calcium and vitamin D are necessary to prevent or overcome rickets.

Rickets is a worse deficiency disease in premature infants because the premie did not have sufficient time to draw enough calcium from the mother. It is only in the last three or four months of pregnancy that the skeleton of a fetus becomes well calcified.

In other instances rickets can arise from poor absorption of vitamin D, as during infection. But a very large intake of cereals can also possibly produce rickets. The reason is that cereals contain a natural material, *phytic acid* or *phytate,* which precipitates calcium; and preventing its absorption makes calcium unavailable.

There is also a vitamin D deficiency in adults, but it does not present the classical picture of rickets. It is a softening and bending of the bone called *osteomalacia,* which may occur in vitamin D deficiency or in pregnancy, when the drain of calcium on the pregnant woman is insuperable. The calcium level of the blood goes down during osteomalacia, indicating the huge extent of calcium impoverishment.

What Does Vitamin D Do?

One cannot speak of vitamin D without speaking of calcium or the parathyroid glands, which control calcium metabolism sparked by vitamin D. Basically, vitamin D allows the absorption of calcium and phosphorus to take place in the intestine. Necessary for development of bone and teeth during growth, it is also needed for maintenance during maturity.

Vitamin D is a fat-soluble vitamin. Hence, in malabsorption there is also impaired absorption of vitamin D, just as there is with vitamins A, E and K. In malabsorption these vitamins are usually given by injection or in water-soluble form.

Food

Vitamin D is usually obtained in foods that are supplemented with it. Milk is fortified with 400 IU of vitamin D, and infant formula preparations and cereals are also supplemented with it because breast milk and nonfortified cow's milk do not contain sufficient amounts.

(See RDA for vitamin D inside front cover.)

BRIEF POINTS ON VITAMIN D

Is deficiency frequent?	No
U.S. RDA?	400 IU
Danger of overdose?	Yes, do not take more than 400 IU daily as supplement.

9

THE ALL-OR-NONE VITAMIN—
VITAMIN E

FOR SOME REASON we cannot fathom, but upon which we can speculate, discussions of vitamin E are surrounded with emotion. There are two camps—those who swear by it and those who swear at it. Both cannot be right. My own opinion is that both are wrong and that we need an assessment without passion—especially since vitamin E does not do a thing in another area of passion, i.e., impotence, for which it was at one time touted.

Vitamin E's first use was to ensure fertility in animals, and about this there is no dispute. Rats have reproductive failure when they are deficient in vitamin E. Then the extrapolation was made to man, and it was promoted as an aphrodisiac. Our Puritan heritage is such that matters connected with sex are furtive, *dirty* and not to be discussed. It would appear that anything that had been offered as an aphrodisiac would thereafter cloud judgment.

The function of vitamin E is that of an antioxidant. An antioxidant protects other substances against oxidation or helps to avert or reduce physiological changes produced by oxidation. Specifically, it acts as an antioxidant in inhibiting or reducing the oxidation of the unsaturated fatty acids of the tissues.

There is no question about the grave events that vitamin E

deficiency produces in animals, with different species of animals showing dysfunction of different organs. Generally vitamin E deficiency shows as reproductive failure in many species, including sterility in the rat and inability to carry the fetus to term. In other animals it can show muscular dystrophy and nutritional dystrophies and degeneration not only of reproductive organs but also of the heart muscle and disturbances of the eyes and other organs.

Obvious signs of deficiency in man develop more slowly. In animals they appear rapidly and dramatically. Although it takes time for signs of deficiency to be clear and recognizable in man, often a year or more, the damage done by deprivation nonetheless occurs. Considering the fact that vitamin E is absorbed through the lymph, is stored in the liver and is found in most organs in man—including kidneys, lungs, pancreas, heart, spleen, liver and muscles, with the highest levels in the adrenal glands, the testes and the pituitary—it becomes apparent how widespread the damage can be through deprivation of vitamin E.

The first sign of a lack of vitamin E may be a certain type of blood destruction which has been reported chiefly in infants; an excess urinary excretion of creatine, a substance involved in muscle contraction, which suggests a metabolic dysfunction in the muscles; or perhaps the deposition of ceroid, an age pigment. But although we do not know, it is possible that the effects of deprivation that give no early signs may be even more serious. There is the danger that by the time symptoms do appear, after a number of years, damage may have already been done in some system.

Deficiency of vitamin E may develop from (1) an inadequate intake, (2) malabsorption, which is reduced ability of the body to absorb fats and vitamin E from the intestine, or (3) an increased intake of polyunsaturated fatty acids.

While deficiency in the human due to inadequate intake of vitamin E is uncommon, clear signs of deficiency occur when vitamin E cannot be utilized. In the malabsorption syndrome deficiency of vitamin E can often occur because then neither vitamin E nor other fat-soluble vitamins—A, D and K—can be absorbed from food.

Vitamin E deficiency can also occur in infants, especially prematures, if there is insufficient intake through the food formula, or because the vitamin E is inactivated by the necessary iron in the formula.

In adults excretion of creatine in the urine, called creatinuria, is a sign that there is something wrong in the metabolism of muscle, and one of several possible dysfunctions may have occurred. Vitamin E has been reported to reverse such creatinuria in many instances. This does *not* mean that vitamin E is the remedy for a variety of muscle dysfunctions.

What Does Vitamin E Do?

A vitamin that is ubiquitous in the human body would appear to have certain functions, even teleologically. Take the case of porphyria. It is not a common disease, yet without a remedy to control it, it raises serious concern. There are different kinds of porphyria. People with porphyria can get abdominal pain that is frequently severe enough to be like a colic, with vomiting and diarrhea, or they can develop psychiatric problems with delusions and hallucinations (such as are said to have been King George III's problems, about which recently theories have been advanced that they were due to porphyria). Or porphyria can affect breathing and cause paralysis of respiration. It can increase pigmentation of the skin, especially after exposure to light, or it can cause a wide distribution of blisters on the skin.

The cause of porphyria is genetic. The disease occurs when nature slips a cog and the individual so affected cannot produce a certain enzyme. The missing enzyme differs with the different kinds of porphyria. But in all of them there is one common trait: certain pigments called porphyrins are overproduced and accumulate in different organs or in the blood. They are also excreted in the urine, but too much remains in the body and creates havoc. Normally, the urine contains only traces of porphyrins.

Although porphyria is rare, when a person gets it it hits him 100 percent. Heretofore, a variety of drugs were used without success—that is, until the stepchild of therapeutics, vitamin E, was tried. Dr. P. P. Nair, director of the biochemistry research division of the department of medicine in the Sinai Hospital of Baltimore, and his associates, Drs. Mezey, Quartner and Murti, are credited with that discovery. A paper published in the September 1971 issue of the highly respected *Archives of Internal Medicine* gives details on several cases and discusses vitamin E and porphyrin metabolism in man.

But you will probably never be faced with treating your porphyria. As a matter of fact you cannot treat it yourself. This brief account is given merely to indicate in a broad view in what areas and corners vitamin E finds a place; and while it does not succeed in some areas, it does in others.

There is no dispute about the nature of vitamin E as an antioxidant. One of the theories about aging is the oxidation theory. This has brought vitamin E into that area. The oxidation theory holds that all things age and become less efficient upon oxidation, which is the chemical process wherein oxygen enters a molecule and changes its structure and function. For example, when a rubber band has become oxidized it loses its elasticity, becomes brittle, and breaks under even a minor stress. The use of vitamin E is based largely on the oxidation theory.

At the Duttweiler Institute Conference on Aging, which met in Zurich, Switzerland, in 1971, great interest was expressed by the participants in various methods to retard the effects of aging. Among other discussions, the greatest thrust was the concern with two antioxidants: (1) butylated hydroxytoluene, which is a chemical used to prevent spoilage of food by oxidation, because it is an antioxidant, and (2) a natural antioxidant, i.e., vitamin E.

Vitamin E has also been reported to protect the organism against the effect of pollution upon the respiratory system. It is reasoned that vitamin E probably protects, against oxidation, the vitamin A which is necessary for the integrity of the mucous membrane of the respiratory tract, as well as the unsaturated fatty acids (lipids) in the tissues of the respiratory tract.

Among other functions, vitamin E protects against the development of blood clots, as described by the world-famous Dr. Alton Ochsner of Tulane University. It improves intermittent claudication, which is a form of circulatory impediment in the legs described by Drs. Williams, Fenna and Macbeth of the University of Alberta Hospital of Edmonton, Alberta, who, using adequate controls, found that that condition improved, but not other circulatory impediments. It remedied a form of anemia of infants which was found by two separate groups of investigators to be due to a vitamin E deficiency: (1) Drs. Ritchie, Fish, McMasters and Grossman of the University of California—San Francisco Medical Center, and (2) Drs. Gross and Guilford of Case Western Reserve University School of Medicine. In short vitamin E acts by stabilizing membranes, guarding them against abnormal breakdown of fat.

A plea for more concentrated study on vitamin E was made by Dr. Knut Naess, who believes that since modern grain-treating methods further reduce our vitamin E intake, intense studies are vital. He holds the view that the vitamin E era has just begun and that we know little about it. The last statement is unquestionably true.

Foods

The following foods are rich in vitamin E: fresh beef liver, wheat germ, fruits and green leafy vegetables, margarine, mayonnaise, nuts, vegetable oils, including corn, peanut and soya oils.

Selenium (see discussion of selenium in Chapter 11) can substitute for some of the effects of vitamin E in certain animals but not, as far as is known, in man.

While polyunsaturated vegetable oils are rich in vitamin E, paradoxically the more unsaturated the oil is, the greater the need for supplementary vitamin E. The reason is that the polyunsaturated oils require vitamin E to protect their own unsaturation.

If taken as a supplement, vitamin E should *not* be used simultaneously with iron because of a mutual incompatibility. If iron is taken in the form of multivitamin-mineral capsules, it may be taken in the morning and vitamin E in the evening, or in any order as long as there is at least a six- to eight-hour span between taking these substances.

(See RDA for vitamin E on inside back cover.)

BRIEF POINTS ON VITAMIN E

U.S. RDA?	30 IU
Danger of overdose?	No

10

THE BLOOD VITAMIN—VITAMIN K

VITAMIN K is the coagulation vitamin—in fact the name vitamin K originates from *Koagulations-Vitamin.*

Under ordinary circumstances vitamin K deficiency does not develop in man, because enough for his needs is made in the small intestine, in addition to which he takes minute amounts in his daily diet. But there are conditions under which deficiency can and does develop. For example, since vitamin K requires bile salts for its utilization, a deficiency of vitamin K can develop if there are insufficient bile salts in the small intestines. That can happen in gallbladder disease or when the elaboration of bile salts is otherwise blocked.

Guarding against hemorrhage, vitamin K allows the blood to clot. It does so by facilitating the synthesis of prothrombin by the liver. Without prothrombin no coagulation of blood can take place (of course, more than prothrombin is involved in the complex mechanism of clotting). But if there is an impairment of liver function it may not be able to manufacture prothrombin, with the result that it will take blood an inordinately long time to clot or hemorrhage can set in. That is the reason why in infectious hepatitis there is a danger of excessive bleeding in case of injury.

Another condition in which vitamin K is not utilized is the

malabsorption syndrome, as the absorption of fat is impeded and vitamin K is a fat-soluble vitamin.

When there is deficiency of vitamin K there are various signs of failure of the blood to clot. An early sign is bleeding areas in the skin (purpura), the common black-and-blue marks after even a mild blow. (This may also be due to vitamin C deficiency.) More serious effects are delayed coagulations or hemorrhage. The possibility of hemorrhage is particularly threatening in the newborn, in the condition called hemorrhagic disease of the newborn. For that reason women about to deliver receive an injection of vitamin K, and newborn babies also usually receive it. The newborn infant needs a few days in order to develop the facility to make its own vitamin K in the intestine. Dr. Herbert I. Goldman reported many instances of puzzling conditions in infants who were found to have only vitamin K deficiency.

There are other events that can influence the destruction of vitamin K, such as the administration antibiotics or sulfonamides. They can kill the bacterial population of the small intestine, so that it cannot produce vitamin K. Diarrhea may be an additional influence which disturbs the life cycle of the bacteria and thereby inhibits vitamin K production in the body.

What Does Vitamin K Do?

It enables blood to clot or prevents its delayed clotting. Hence, it prevents and treats the hemorrhagic disease of the newborn. Milk substitutes for infants are now fortified with small amounts of vitamin K.

The function of vitamin K is not limited to the newborn. It aids in wound healing—a bleeding wound does not heal. That is the reason it is given after surgery if the vitamin K level in the blood is low. But this is useful only if the bleeding is due to vitamin K deficiency or inadequate synthesis of prothrombin. Other conditions are also operative in blood coagulation.

In the alcoholic, the probability of excessive bleeding is increased since his liver, probably impaired, is not functioning adequately. Hence it cannot use vitamin K efficiently in the production of prothrombin. A cirrhotic liver is like a factory that is half shut down and therefore cannot produce its proper output.

Vitamin K is often needed by people who are receiving anticoagulants. If the dose of anticoagulant is too high, or other drugs taken have exaggerated the anticoagulant effect, the prothrombin time is increased and this may possibly lead to bleeding. At such a time, vitamin K is given usually by injection.

Food

The vitamin K we need is usually adequately supplied in our food intake and by the intestinal bacteria which synthesize it in man. It is found in nature in green leafy vegetables. Certain chemicals have vitamin K activity; they are called vitamins K_1, K_2 and K_3. While vitamin K is a fat-soluble vitamin, water-soluble derivatives have been made. They are particularly necessary for injection during bleeding episodes.

The richest sources of vitamin K are green leafy vegetables, pork liver, cows' milk, and vegetable oils. Supplementation is usually not necessary since sufficient is available between the natural production in the intestine and the small intake in food. Extraordinary circumstances that require supplementation, such as the conditions previously described, should be treated by a physician.

11

THE MICRONUTRIENTS
(TRACE METALS, TRACE MINERALS,
TRACE ELEMENTS)

What Are the Micronutrients?

WINE WAS USED as a high-voltage social lubricant for thousands of years. Religious cults were often built around wine. The word *dionysiac* which has come down into our language originated from the cult of Dionysus, or Bacchus, in which wine was the central point uniting the communicants. Orgies float on rivers of wine.

Then, more than a hundred years ago, a great discovery was made. Wine which had been allowed to stand in rusty iron pails was used as a medicine. If it did not work as a medicine, at least if taken in quantity it dulled the troubles that ailed you. The rusty containers had naturally added iron to the wine. When people learned that secret they refined the technique: a few rusty nails were just soaked in the wine; after a generous intake of that medicine the user was also soaked.

Thus, in contaminating wine, iron became a medicine. Why, then, was there no progress made until recently in determining which of the trace minerals, metals, elements or micronutrients are essential for man or other animals? Simply because being distributed merely in traces or in such minute amounts, no analytical methods were sensitive enough to determine a concentration of only a few parts per million. And only such minute amounts are necessary for well-being.

While the vitamins are of animal or vegetable origin, the micronutrients and minerals, as their name implies, are of mineral origin. Many are indispensable in nutrition, in fact to health itself; they are found in the crust of the earth, also in the seas, in fact everywhere on earth. The reason they are referred to as *trace minerals* is one of quantity: the trace minerals or micronutrients are needed in minute amounts, often sheer traces, while other minerals like calcium are needed in larger amounts. Another name for trace minerals is *trace elements* or *trace metals*. Recently they have been called the *micronutrients* or *inorganic micronutrients*. All these names are synonymous. We will refer to them mostly as *micronutrients*.

Those now known to be essential for man are chromium, cobalt, copper, manganese, molybdenum, selenium and zinc. (These are not listed in order of importance, merely alphabetically.) The following may possibly also be found soon to be essential trace minerals: silicon, tin and vanadium. Magnesium, though necessary in comparatively larger amounts—i.e., about 400 mg per day —is still considered a trace mineral. (There are other minerals— calcium, sodium, potassium, etc.—which are also essential but they are not considered to be trace minerals.)

There are about twenty other minerals which are not, or not yet found to be, essential to human nutrition. Further research may determine if they are. Here is a partial alphabetical list: aluminum, antimony, arsenic, barium, boron, bromine, cadmium, gallium, lead, lithium, mercury, nickel, rubidium, silver, strontium and titanium. About thirty or forty more were reported to be found in living organisms, including plants and microorganisms.

In fact, the impetus for determining whether a given micronutrient is essential to man was originally based on the fact that it was found in living organisms. The reasoning here is teleological: if nature put it there, it must have a purpose. But there are so many exceptions to that concept. One example: Dr. Henry Schroeder, to whom we owe most of the fundamental information on micronutrients, found that lead is widely distributed in nature and found in human tissues in minute amounts as well as in the tissues of wild animals which are not exposed to industrial contaminants. On the basis of that concept, one can infer that lead is an essential micronutrient; probably it is not. Lead, like cadmium, another poisonous metal, inhibits and often destroys an enzyme system. A similar situation may apply to titanium. It is found in most foods consumed by man, accumulates in the lungs, but it has little if any biological activity. While it is not believed to be toxic, it is probably not an essential micronutrient.

Micronutrient needs in man, and those needed by other animals and plants, are not necessarily the same. Many plants, for example, require boron while man apparently does not. But plants and many animals all need copper, iron, manganese, molybdenum and zinc.

Several fascinating characteristics are applicable to micronutrients:

1. They are effective or utilizable in minute quantities, as, for example, 1 microgram of cobalt, as part of the B_{12} molecule (but not by itself) can control pernicious anemia (a microgram is a millionth of a gram and there are 28.35 grams to the ounce). But continuing intake of 3 micrograms of a poisonous mineral, say, cadmium, if retained, can be toxic.

2. You cannot live without an essential micronutrient, and an inadequate intake can produce deficiency symptoms.

3. Excessive amounts of some micronutrients can kill, as, for example, selenium.

4. A deficiency can become more serious in the presence of such stresses as exposure, growth, pregnancy, surgery or disease.

5. There is an interrelationship among micronutrients with each other and with the metabolic environment. For example, excessive zinc in rats can inhibit growth and produce anemia, but that is overcome by increased intake of copper; or too much manganese can inhibit the synthesis of hemoglobin; or too much zinc, nickel or manganese in sheep interferes with their storage of copper. In man, the administration of magnesium can increase calcium excretion. Other examples of antagonism among micronutrients are plentiful.

6. With certain exceptions, the body has a low storage ability for micronutrients, but unfortunately that is more true of the "good" micronutrients than of poisonous ones; an example is the cumulation of lead—a bad guy—which can produce lead poisoning.

7. Signs of deficiency are clearer in other animals than in man. There are several reasons for this: (a) it is easy to starve them; (b) they are expendable; (c) growth and life-span in most animals are shorter than in man, hence the effects of deprivations are more prominent or concentrated due to their rapid growth rate and more critical demands within a shorter period of time. Man's more complex and varied food intake probably makes deficiencies of certain micronutrients more rare but they are more likely to occur during periods of stress. Man's more complex metabolism can have a "sparing effect," which means a "little can go a longer way," because another substance may partially substitute for it.

8. Certain minerals needed in other animals, such as silicon or tin, may not be necessary in man, or perhaps man obtains the infinitesimal quantities he needs quite adventitiously, like a trace of tin from his use of canned food.

Dr. Henry Schroeder, to whom and to whose associates we owe much of what we know about micronutrients, states that they are more important than vitamins, because some vitamins can be synthesized by the body but micronutrients cannot be at all and must be obtained from the environment. While man can indeed synthesize vitamin K in his gut and vitamin D in his skin, he must obtain most other vitamins from his environment as, unlike other animals, he cannot synthesize them in his body. For example, he cannot synthesize vitamin A or vitamin C.

Deficiency

But deficiency of micronutrients conceivably can occur in man. One reason may be eccentric or fanatic diets. Another is severe malnutrition such as found in overpopulated and economically deprived parts of the world. We will discuss additional reasons under the separate micronutrients. Unless, as in zinc, the damage is irreversible, taking the micronutrients will overcome deficiency signs, and continuing to take them will protect against deficiency signs appearing.

The determination about a given micronutrient is firmly based upon the following chain of events. First, a diet is fed which contains all known food elements except the one in which the researcher is interested to find out whether it is essential. Second, he looks for deficiency symptoms which must arise. Third, he investigates whether deficiency symptoms are reversed when the missing micronutrient is fed.

While this is a proper and logical scientific procedure it allows a logical fallacy to creep in. Science usually lies in wait to befuddle the researcher. Here is what can happen: a deficiency symptom may not be reversible. That surely will pull the rug out from under the well-designed experiment. Had sufficient micronutrients been available, such an irreversible deficiency symptom would not have occurred.

Here is an illustration: in vitamin A deficiency, certain symptoms of eye dysfunction occur, such as vision impairment in twilight. This is reversed by vitamin A. So far so good. However, in profound vitamin A deficiency the child so deprived may become blind. And blindness is not reversible. So if vitamin A were to be administered to a child who was blind because of severe vitamin A deficiency, the child would not regain sight. Hence, the way we now assess the essential nature of a micronutrient (and vitamins as well), it can well be reasoned that vitamin A is not an essential vitamin because it did not give the child back its sight; thus blindness is not a deficiency symptom. But this is the best method we now have of testing whether a micronutrient or a vitamin is an essential one.

These experiments are done on animals, notably on rats. While findings in these animals do largely apply to man it is not at all certain that the finding in one species of animal is applicable to other species. Only effects observed in man can clearly apply to man, and even in the same species there are notable exceptions. We call these exceptions *biological individuality* because we do not understand them. At least that tables the question for a moment while we are trying to figure out the answer.

Mineral Overload

Too much of a good thing can be bad and that applies to gorging on micronutrients as well as on goodies. You will recall among the attributes of a micronutrient that (a) it is essential in small quantities, (b) it can be poisonous in excess. With micronutrients, and in fact with other minerals as well, an overload can be dangerous. This does not mean that the micronutrients or mineral tablets available in drugstores or health food stores are dangerous—they are not. At worst they may not be well balanced or the form of the mineral used may not be available to or utilizable by the body, but they are not toxic.

An example of a micronutrient that may be toxic is selenium. *Do not take supplementary selenium.* Depend on the selenium in certain foods that are safely rich in it; these are enumerated later in the section on selenium.

Another example of a mineral that might be overloaded is iron. Iron is an essential mineral but too much in certain people can raise trouble. (See the section on iron.) Copper overload can also occur. Here is how excessive intake of minerals or micronutrients can possibly take place:

1. Incredibly huge intake of otherwise safe foods or mineral supplement tablets.

2. Through cooking utensils—especially applicable to copper or iron utensils.

3. Tremendous intake of water—this is especially applicable in tropical climates where an immense amount of water is drunk and a gigantic amount of water is lost through perspiration; the water itself is "sweated out" but the minerals or micronutrients in which the water may be rich build up cumulatively in the body.

4. Excessive absorption or utilization by the body of even a moderate mineral intake due to an inborn error in metabolism where nature *slipped a cog* and did not provide a given enzyme, used in the conversion or excretion of a mineral or micronutrient. An example would be iron-storage disease.

5. Low protein intake—many minerals require proteins for their proper metabolic conversion.

6. Alcoholism, which includes drinking beer, since the volume of liquid consumed can be considerable. Some prac-

tices in brewing, especially among certain African tribes (Bantus), produce beer with a high proportion of iron in the final product due to the iron vessels used in brewing. This, accentuated by the effects of alcohol, which is a liver poison, coupled with a low-protein diet, sets the stage for the inability of the body to absorb or excrete iron efficiently, which thus builds up.

7. Increased iron absorption due to the body's compensatory mechanism to absorb more of a substance when more is needed. For example, the absorption of iron by the body is increased in iron-deficiency anemia (and in no other type of anemia); this can happen during pregnancy or growth; ordinarily, excess iron would be excreted.

But nearly all of the preceding conditions are rare.

You need not fear developing iron overload or an overload of other micronutrients through food, even if you take large amounts. It would take pounds and pounds of spinach or dried apricots consumed at one sitting and used frequently to develop such an overload. Nor is there likelihood of developing iron or other mineral overload in taking mineral supplements, unless you take 10 to 25 times or more the usual amounts given on the label. In other words, even a heavy diet, within reason, will not overload anything but your stomach.

Here, too, an exception can arise. If the proposed enrichment of bread with iron becomes a reality, it may well happen that people who have iron-storage disease (see section on iron) and who consume inordinately large amounts of bread may possibly suffer detrimental effects from iron.

What Do Micronutrients Do?

Briefly, they activate enzyme systems in the body. There are thousands of enzyme reactions which make the totality of life.

Magnesium, for example, is an integral part of the energy enzyme system called the adenosine triphosphate or ATP system, enabling variants to release energy for every function of life, pick it up again, and repeat the cycle endlessly. When that cycle ceases, life ends.

How Essential Are the Micronutrients?

Many researchers believe that even by the spotty evidence now available the micronutrients may have a greater role in development of chronic diseases than we now imagine. This is entirely reasonable when we see the findings in subsequent sections.

Dr. Walter Mertz, chief of the Agricultural Research Service of the U.S. Department of Agriculture in Beltsville, Maryland, who is also editor of the authoritative book *Trace Elements in Nutrition,* and Dr. Harold Sandstead, director of the Human Nutrition Laboratory of the Agricultural Research Service of the U.S. Department of Agriculture in Grand Forks, North Dakota, point out that the micronutrients are available only in small quantities *even with a very good diet,* and except for a few, the body does not have an efficient way of storing them for future use. Hence, they believe that a deficiency can take place at some stage between intake and utilization.

Another factor enters: the need for certain micronutrients increases with age and in the presence of certain disease conditions, as diabetes. Supplementation by chromium helps relieve diabetes. Drs. Mertz and Sandstead recommend that physicians should familiarize themselves with those micronutrients that up to now were considered exotic—namely, chromium, manganese, molybdenum, selenium and zinc, as these have a fundamental role in health and disease because they are enzyme activators.

Drs. Mertz and Sandstead hold that the ordinary dietary intake does not assure an optimum supply of micronutrients, especially in illness. Nonetheless they recommend a balanced diet which includes both meat and vegetables as a source because we do not know precisely how much is needed for average daily use of most micronutrients. They remind us that processing reduces the amount of micronutrients—as, for example, flour milling removes from whole wheat 80 percent of zinc and iron, 88 percent of manganese and 62 percent of molybdenum. An extraordinary thing takes place in the milling process: while milling removes a substantial part of these micronutrients it also destroys phytic acid.

Phytic acid is the simple name for the jawbreaking chemical inositolhexaphosphoric acid. A name like that sticks to the tongue more than milled flour. Phytic acid is not a good thing because it binds certain minerals, notably zinc and probably other micronutrients, and makes them unavailable.

A short explanation of chemical binding should be helpful here: micronutrients are usually combined with certain proteins in the course of metabolism but then must be freed from the binding in order to be utilized by the body. Some proteins keep a loose bond with the micronutrients and give them up easily. Others, like phytic acid, make a tight bond and do not give them up readily. A substance is considered unavailable if it is tightly bound with a protein and cannot enter into the metabolic reactions in the body for good nutrition. Other words for *unavailable* are *unutilizable* or *insoluble,* but those may lead to an ambiguous understanding.

Now, while milling removes valuable micronutrients it also destroys the phytic acid or phytate, leaving what little of the micronutrients that are left free from bondage to phytate. It may be a case of six of one and half a dozen of another—we don't know yet.

But what does this mean to the individual concerned with good nutrition: especially, should he be devoted to whole wheat and other "natural" products from which micronutrients have not been extracted? It means that in the imperfect state of our knowledge it would appear that one can be both on foot and on horseback or, to use another metaphor, he can have the best of two imperfect worlds by including in his diet *both* whole wheat products and enriched white bread.

Here is another illustration of binding which does not have anything to do with nutrition: carbon monoxide kills because it tightly binds hemoglobin in the blood and does not give up its oxygen readily. Hence the oxygen becomes unavailable. Hemoglobin, on the other hand, has a loose binding with oxygen; hemoglobin is like an oxygen sponge taking in oxygen copiously from which it can be easily wrung out, thus making oxygen available for respiration.

Hemoglobin is a protein-metal complex that binds oxygen loosely, and on it our breathing and our life depend. The tightly bound protein-metal complex is called carboxyhemoglobin, and it holds oxygen in a death-grip.

Phytic acid is called a chelating agent, which is a substance that has a firm grip on a substance that comes in contact with it and does not easily release it. This can be better understood by noting that the word chelation comes from the Greek *kylos,* meaning a claw.

While certain micronutrients serve a critical function in the life and work of enzymes (see Chapter 14 on enzymes), they have other functions as well, which we suspect but do not yet understand. Micronutrients facilitate enzyme function. Some proteins are enzymes. When micronutrients are bound to a protein that is an enzyme (metal-enzyme complex) they facilitate the functioning of that enzyme. Thus micronutrients such as cobalt, copper, iron, magnesium, manganese, molybdenum, nickel and zinc activate or spark the function of certain enzyme systems, i.e., they make them *whole* enzymes. (Every enzyme is a protein but not every protein is an enzyme.)

The same micronutrients, and perhaps others as well, are bound to nucleic acids (RNA and DNA), which are also of fundamental importance to well-being—in fact, to life.

Micronutrients have also been studied with varied degrees of intensity to determine if they have a role in aging, in either retarding or hastening the deteriorating effect of age, physical or mental. Their role in other diseases is also being investigated. The future should produce some probative evidence of their role in aging because recently several highly sensitive methods of analysis have been developed which can determine the minute traces in which the micronutrients occur.

Heart

A number of micronutrients have a relationship to the functions of the heart. At the fifth annual Conference on Trace Minerals in Environmental Health held at the University of Missouri in August 1971, it was reported that copper, manganese and zinc (together with vitamins C and E as well as estrogens and thyroid) reduced the occurrence of a second heart attack in controlled groups of people who had survived one heart attack. Other effects of micronutrients in heart function were reported by Drs. D'Alonzo and Pell—as, for example, magnesium reducing fat in blood vessels, which is associated with heart attacks. Cholesterol is one such fatty material. A micronutrient, vanadium, has been reported to inhibit cholesterol synthesis by the body. The findings of other investigators seem to take another tack, in that they found that the levels of other micronutrients, as boron, molybdenum and nickel, are high in patients who have suffered a heart attack.

One of the great questions and disputes still raging concerns soft water. Water is considered soft when it is relatively free from calcium and magnesium. Soft water is reported by some to cause hardening of the arteries or arteriosclerosis. (*Arteriosclerosis* is the hardening of the arteries in aging. *Atherosclerosis* is something else; not limited to any age group, it is a building up within the blood vessels of a layer of lipids or fats, notably cholesterol, which impedes the circulation of the blood in the vessels.)

For example, Dr. Terence W. Anderson of the University of Toronto stated at the International Water Quality Symposium in Washington, D.C., that it is quite probable that soft water is a considerable factor in the development of arteriosclerosis. This idea was first brought up by Dr. Henry Schroeder, the pioneer in the study of micronutrients. More recently, Drs. Stitt, Crawford, Clayton and Morris of the London School of Hygiene and Tropical Medicine took a much more positive view in the eminent British medical journal *Lancet* of January 20, 1973. They conducted a controlled experiment in which 244 men living in hard-water towns and 245 in soft-water towns participated. They found that in men living in soft-water towns, blood pressure, cholesterol levels and heart rate were higher. These signs usually prepare the soil for a heart attack.

Micronutrients in the water supply have several origins. Part is derived from decaying vegetation as some plants selectively concentrate given minerals. Another source is the natural chemical erosion or chemical weathering of the soil, or the soluble products of soil formation.

Arthritis

New ideas and new substances are more likely to be first tried in diseases that are still puzzling—arthritis and cancer, to name two. The role of micronutrients was studied in both of them. One type of arthritis, rheumatoid arthritis, is a serious and usually disabling disease unless it is under control or its symptoms are in remission. Hence, almost anything is worthy of study in rheumatoid arthritis. Dr. William Niedermeiser, assistant professor of medicine at the University of Alabama, studied the level of micronutrients in the *joint fluid* of patients with rheumatoid arthritis and found that aluminum, barium, cadmium (the last two are poisonous metals), strontium and tin were lower than normal, but the following were higher: copper and zinc three times as high and iron twice as high as the levels normally found. But in the *blood serum* iron and zinc levels were lower. This suggests that higher or lower levels are not necessarily related to rheumatoid arthritis, but that there is a derangement of the micronutrients in that condition. What it is due to or what it really means is not known.

Cancer

It would be expected that the role of micronutrients would be studied in cancer. While findings do not tell a clear story, additional insights have been gained which need further study. One important finding is that platinum compounds inhibit certain cancers in mice (leukemia and sarcoma). Whether that applies to man is not yet known. But a more important finding is that *platinum and palladium increase the effect of anticancer drugs.* (Leukemia is cancer of the bone marrow; sarcoma is cancer that can occur in various tissues such as muscle, bone fatty tissue, nerve and cartilage.)

Other findings of levels of micronutrients in cancers: copper, magnesium, manganese, tin and zinc are lower in some cancerous tissue than in corresponding noncancerous tissue. But zinc is higher in cancerous tissue of the lung than in the noncancerous.

What does this mean in relation to cancer? Very little, but the pieces of the jigsaw puzzle may make a picture with further research.

Man is uncomfortable with ambiguities and uncertainties. Therefore, he often jumps to conclusions and sprains an intellectual ankle doing so. Applied to micronutrients, it does not mean that because a high level of certain micronutrients was found in a given disease, it is a cause of that disease or even a result of it. That applies, too, when a low level of a certain micronutrient is found in a given condition. It merely means that such-or-such an abnormality is associated with the disease, in the group being studied. While one cannot and should not conclude cause-and-effect relationships, such an abnormality suggests an opening. Many more confirmatory studies are necessary in a variety of different populations before one is entitled even to hold an opinion, and surely before a conclusion can justifiably be drawn. In science, conclusions can be tentative for a long time.

In the following sections each of the micronutrients is briefly described as to what it has been found to do and often what happens in the body in case of deficiency. They are arranged alphabetically and not in order of importance; all of them are important for different reasons.

CADMIUM

Better let your faucet run before you take a drink, because galvanized pipes contain cadmium. It is known that cadmium inactivates certain enzymes. It is otherwise believed to be a poisonous micronutrient, and Schroeder believes it increases the incidence of high blood pressure and, hence, heart disease. He believes that it comes into food as a minute contaminant from galvanized water pipes or from the plating of ice cube trays, in the manufacture of which cadmium has been used in the past. He reasons that cadmium standing in galvanized pipes and in the newer black plastic pipes can be leached out from them, aided by slight acidity of water, and therefore recommends letting some water run out before using it in food or for drinking. Other investigators have confirmed Dr. Schroeder's findings and believe that though cadmium may not be the sole responsible factor in high blood pressure, its presence triggers it in people who are constitutionally so disposed.

The highest amounts of cadmium were found by Schroeder in sea food, especially in oysters, both fresh and canned, crabmeat, lobster, shrimp; also in canned salmon, tuna and anchovies, and fresh swordfish. Certain grains, especially flour, and canned fruit juices (lemon, pineapple, tomato, due to their high acid content) have also been found high in cadmium.

Cadmium poisoning occurs more frequently among Japanese, in whom a condition called "ouch, ouch disease" occurs. This was found to be due to chronic cadmium poisoning, derived from environmental pollution. The term "ouch, ouch" is a translation of the Japanese "itai, itai," which is its equivalent expletive. People who have the disease cry out "itai, itai" upon being touched, as their joints and back are extremely painful, and bone fractures occur easily. The reason may be that cadmium drains calcium from the tissues, including bone.

Cadmium does occur naturally in certain wild animal tissue (liver and kidney), but whether it fills a biological role is not known. It may be merely an environmental contaminant. The chances are that it has no biological role to play.

Do not take cadmium as a supplement.

CHROMIUM

Long used in metal plating it was discovered only as recently as 1959 that chromium activates insulin action. Insulin plays a vital role in carbohydrate or glucose utilization during a state of well-being and even more in diabetes, in which there is a disarrangement of carbohydrate or glucose metabolism. In fact, a combination of chromium with a body protein is actually called GTF —glucose tolerance factor. (But do not assume that chromium is the whole story in the diabetes-insulin relationship; it is only one, though an important, part.)

The same Drs. Mertz and Sandstead previously mentioned originally found the role of chromium as the glucose tolerance factor in diabetes in animals and man. Their work was repeated in diabetic patients by Dr. R. A. Levine of the Upstate Medical Center in Syracuse, who observed an improvement in his diabetic patients after giving them chromium supplements. Another condition, such as kwashiorkor, the disfiguring and killing protein-poverty disease in children, was also improved by chromium administration. This does not mean that chromium stands in place of rehabilitation with other nutrients.

Chromium levels in the body are depleted with age, which is unfortunate, as this is just the time when the incidence of degenerative diseases rises. Since even good diets do not supply an adequate amount of chromium, according to Drs. Mertz and Sandstead, they consider supplementation a wise move. They base this on the premise that there is a mild deficiency of chromium in the older population of the United States.

Dr. Schroeder first studied chromium in 1960; at that time he suspected it to be an essential micronutrient, which has since been accepted. Another of his findings, in animals, that chromium reduced cholesterol in the blood has since been confirmed clinically. Schroeder was the first to report (among his other "firsts") that the chromium content of the aorta of people who died of heart attack was lower than that of those who died accidentally. This suggests strongly that chromium may be one influence in the protection against heart attack for one reason at least, i.e., because it may act on fat metabolism, reducing it.

The following foods are highest in a useful form of chromium: corn oil, black pepper, thyme, brewers' yeast, mushrooms, beef liver, bread. Various forms of refinement and milling of foods also remove chromium. Urine is a rich source of chromium, which is no solace, but it merely means that the kidneys excrete chromium. Refined sugar increases chromium excretion.

Chromium can be toxic—it has been to workers exposed to relatively high concentration for long periods of time. Another toxic effect of chromium in factories using it in metal plating or in making dyes is an ulceration of the nasal tissues when it is inhaled. That is another form of chromium—not the form used in supplementation.

Do not take supplemental chromium unless your doctor prescribes it.

COBALT

When a group of beer drinkers in Quebec began to drop dead it caused great consternation. People were warned against the dissolute life of drinking beer. It strengthened their own feelings of sanctimoniousness. Soon it was evident that the deaths were local, though sporadic reports came from the western part of Canada. That was because the Quebec beer was shipped there.

Similar incidents were also reported in Omaha, Nebraska. The cause was suspected to be cobalt. In these two cities the brewers added appreciable amounts of a cobalt salt because it gave beer a much better "head" (foam) while it conked out hearts and livers of previously healthy beer drinkers.

There is no doubt now that the deaths were due to the added cobalt, for when the brewers stopped adding it, there were no more deaths. Whether the poisoning by cobalt was compounded by malnutrition and the lessened resistance due to alcohol is not known. But it is known that the drinkers who died succumbed not only to considerable heart enlargement but also to liver involvement—the badge of alcoholism.

Compare that with the saving of lives from pernicious anemia and tropical sprue through the use of vitamin B_{12}. What does vitamin B_{12} have to do with cobalt? Everything. It owes its effect to cobalt, which is a component of vitamin B_{12}. In fact, vitamins B_{12} are called *cobalamins*. Two substances, cyanocobalamin and hydroxycobalamin, are, in fact, vitamin B_{12}.

Cobalt also stimulates the production of red blood cells in many animals. It can do so overgenerously and is not used in man for that purpose. A most important function of cobalt is as a metallic component in several enzyme systems which convert enzymes into forms probably necessary in cell metabolism.

Cobalt, obtained by man through animal materials in his diet, is found in liver, kidneys and bones. A diet containing a moderate amount of meat probably supplies the small amount needed. That is another reason why the skewed diets of vegetarians lack nutritional wisdom.

Do not take cobalt as a supplement unless your doctor recommends it.

COPPER

Paradoxical indeed—though copper deficiency has not been reported in man, the need for copper in human nutrition is imperative. Enough is probably found in the diet. Certain diseases increase the copper level in the blood, with unfortunate results, probably because they hold back its excretion. Conversely, when the copper level is low it is probably due to increased excretion.

Yet, the relation may not be as simple as that because there is a dynamic interrelationship among the micronutrients. One micronutrient can cause a deficiency in another, as well as a superabundance. For example, too much of another micronutrient, molybdenum, can produce a deficiency of copper, because by making copper insoluble it blocks its uptake and utilization by the body. Extra copper remedies it. Zinc, another micronutrient, is also antagonistic to copper.

There is a liver disease, Wilson's disease, in which an excess of copper accumulates in the liver and causes liver and nerve degeneration. This is a metabolic error, a genetic condition whereby nature "slipped a cog," and prevents the natural function of enzymes to keep the myriad body functions in balance.

While copper deficiency is not reported in man except in rare instances, in malnourished babies there do exist other conditions in which there is copper deficiency. *Kinky-hair syndrome* is found in certain infants in whom there is copper deficiency due to metabolic error. The hair is sparse and incredibly kinky. The most impressive research on copper as a micronutrient and its role in health and disease was done by Drs. M. M. Wintrobe and George E. Cartwright at the University of Utah.

Copper probably has a role in blood formation and may be involved in the degeneration of blood vessels; certain research may confirm this. Other experimental evidence suggests that copper and zinc together may reduce lipids in blood, as cholesterol.

In the body, copper is normally stored in the liver and in a circulating protein in blood called ceruloplasmin. Its level in the blood is normally steady except that it may be low in the newborn. An enzyme is needed to utilize it. In Wilson's disease, previously mentioned, copper is high in the tissues but low in the circulating blood from which it is utilized by the body. It is interesting to note that with aging copper increases in the brain but decreases in many other organs, as the liver, lung and spleen.

The daily requirement is about 2 mg, about one-tenth that of iron. In fact, in early times when iron was effectively used in hypochromic anemia it may have been more effective because copper was a contaminant in the iron.

Copper is found in beef liver, oysters, peas and nuts. The U.S. RDA for copper is 2 mg.

FLUORINE

Part bug-killer and part dental guardian against caries, fluorine is an excellent example of one of the characteristics of micronutrients: too little can create severe deficiency symptoms and too much can be toxic.

Fluorine is well known as an additive to toothpastes and to drinking water in the proportion of 1 ppm (1 part per million). This protects against dental caries in childhood and adolescence and its desirable effect extends to adulthood. The range of 5 ppm can be toxic.

Too much fluorine can lead to a mottling of teeth and fragility of the tooth enamel. It can also produce a generalized hardening of all the bony structures of the body. This very quality is judiciously utilized in the treatment of osteoporosis, which is a softening of bone due to loss of calcium. The bone loses much of its substance, becoming less dense. Calcium, the mineral that is the bony "filler" or support of bone, migrates out of bone and deposits into the tissues. Osteoporosis is a gradual process beginning in about the forties and increasing during aging. This is one reason for increased incidence of fractures among older people because their bones lose density and strength. Certain cortisonelike drugs can also produce osteoporosis.

It is in osteoporosis—whether due to aging or to taking adrenal corticosteroids (cortisonelike drugs)—that fluorine has been recently used. The objective was to support the bony structure, to reduce resorption or bone loss, and to stimulate bone formation by a crystalline growth in bone that is more stable. This work was recently described by Dr. Daniel S. Bernstein and his associates of Harvard Medical School, by Dr. Clayton Rich, Jr., of the Veterans Administration Hospital of Seattle, and by Dr. Jenifer Jowsoy and her associates of the Mayo Clinic, among others. The whole idea is to support and strengthen bone and hopefully to prevent migration of calcium into the larger blood vessels, which is tantamount to arteriosclerosis.

Fluoride may work both by retaining calcium in bone and by forming a firmer *crystalline structure* of bone. (The strength of many solid substances, including bone, depends largely on the size, shape and arrangement of microscopic crystals, referred to generally as crystalline structure.) While fluorine stimulates bone formation, it requires calcium and vitamin D for its function. But the whole story of how fluorine works in this area is not fully understood.

The term *fluorine* is the element itself; *fluoride* is its combination with sodium or calcium, in which form it is found in nature and utilized by the body. Fluorine exists in most foodstuffs (as fluoride), seafoods and tea being especially rich in it. Milk also contains a small amount of fluoride, but it is not in a soluble, hence not in an available, form.

We speak of 1 ppm fluorine in water as being optimum, but that depends largely on how much water is consumed and especially how much food high in fluorine, such as seafood or tea, is consumed. That is difficult to determine. But no deficiency of fluorine, except in caries, has been found. On the contrary, excessive intake is often the case—as, for example, in the Punjab region of India, the water in some localities contains the immensely high proportion of 15 ppm. In addition to the large amount in the water in the Punjab there is a high water intake due to the hot climate and its continuous loss from the body through perspiration. It is amazing that there is no epidemic poisoning with such a high intake.

Do not take fluorine as a supplement. When used for osteoporosis it must be ordered by a physician who has the experience and facilities to monitor its intake. But there is no objection to the regular use of fluoride-containing toothpastes.

IODINE

Iodine is needed for protection against goiter and for the normal functions of the thyroid gland. It is an essential micronutrient. Iodized salt is a good form in which to assure the necessary intake of iodine. At times, however, especially on salt-restricted diets, it is necessary to take iodine in other forms which can usually be recommended by a physician.

Iodine is necessary throughout life, but its need is perhaps somewhat greater during pregnancy, lactation and adolescence.

Seafood, spinach and kelp are rich in iodine, as are cod and haddock among salt-water fish. By contrast, iodine is only moderately present in fresh-water fish and in vegetables other than the above. Diets rich in soybeans definitely require supplemental iodine since they contain a substance which is said to be *goitrogenic*—namely, goiter-producing, by reducing the uptake of iodine. This can be overcome by a small additional supplement of iodine, as in iodized salt. It should be borne in mind that while soybean is a good source of protein, heating converts it into a more utilizable form.

The U.S. RDA of iodine is 150 micrograms.

IRON

The iron heart is a weak heart. But iron is vital for many functions.

That small percentage of the population with iron-storage disease can suffer damage from iron. Those who have another condition called hemochromatosis, in which the tissues are stained with hemoglobin or other blood pigments, are also exposed to hazards of iron. The cirrhotic liver of alcoholics (Laennec's cirrhosis) normally has an uphill task to handle the hundreds of normal detoxifications to support life; iron adds considerably to its burden. In Cooley's anemia (also called thalassemia), iron may disturb the precarious blood balance by further enlarging the liver, in which organ much of the iron is stored.

The iron heart is a weak heart according to Drs. Buja and Roberts in an article in the August 1971 issue of the *American Journal of Medicine*. Of 135 patients, of whom only 4 had hemochromatosis and 131 had chronic anemia, 19 had deposits of iron in the heart. When there is an iron deposit in the heart, the heart fails. The excess iron in these people came from blood transfusions, and since nearly all of them had anemia, probably from excessive iron medications.

Making iron available is one thing. Utilizing it is another. For example, people with low stomach acidity (hypochlorhydria) cannot utilize iron adequately. But the administration of vitamin C helps the utilization of iron in normal individuals as well as those with hypochlorhydria.

Iron is not the safe substance it is commonly thought to be for another reason—mineral overload is possible with too much iron.

More iron does not necessarily mean "better blood." It does not even mean better absorption, because there is an extraordinary balance that the body observes: the more supplemental iron that is taken *when not needed*, the less efficient the absorption. Conversely, in iron-deficiency anemia there is an avid absorption of what iron is available and utilizable.

The foregoing are the negative aspects of iron, mentioned to give an adequate picture of its advantages and disadvantages, especially to a segment of the population to which it can be toxic. Yet iron is a vital substance and iron deficiency is a real and widespread problem, possibly one of the most widespread throughout the world. You cannot live without iron.

Iron is vitally necessary in the daily diet. The U.S. Ten-State Nutrition Survey, reporting that low levels of iron are widespread, also found that many diets were deficient in iron content.

Iron deficiency gives rise to such symptoms as lassitude, breathlessness and weakness, and in severe instances the heart may be affected and even edema can set in. The heart can suffer from too much iron and definitely from too little. This is largely due to the reduction of hemoglobin, and thereby insufficient oxygen is carried to the tissues for respiratory and other functions. (There is also a form of anemia due to both iron and zinc deficiency—see zinc.)

Iron-deficiency anemia can result from one or more of a number of events:

1. The obvious one is lack of sufficient dietary intake of iron and in infants a lack of iron supplementation.
2. Even if the iron intake is sufficient there may be a malabsorption of iron, i.e., poor absorption or assimilation, such as in older people when there is not enough hydrochloric acid in the stomach.
3. Blood loss may have occurred due to trauma, excessive menstruation, surgery or obstetric delivery, and this would occasion loss of iron.
4. Or loss of iron may be due to hidden bleeding (occult blood loss), as in hemorrhoids, or bleeding from the intestines, which is not easily noticeable.

Iron is needed during periods of growth, menstruation, pregnancy and especially during lactation and after delivery, due to either increased need for iron or undue loss of blood. It is also needed by aging people who, due to dietary eccentricities or economic need, are likely to have a diet deficient in iron.

Not all iron is the same—in other words not all iron is equally available, utilizable and absorbable. One of the reasons is that it may be bound to a protein that does not readily release it. Normally, iron is bound to a substance called *transferin*, which is a blood protein but which readily releases iron, i.e., it *transfers iron*. Iron bound to certain foods by phytates, as in cereals or eggs, or oxalates in spinach, is not easily available iron.

The availability or absorbability of iron is enhanced by an acid food or medium, especially by vitamin C, which is ascorbic acid. Dr. Sheila T. Callender reports, for example, that orange juice increases the absorption of iron from eggs. And the absorbability of iron from meat is superior to that from vegetables.

Iron fumarate is a good source of iron if taken as a supplement.

Spinach as the traditionally rich source of iron bears reexamination. According to the Vitamin Information Bureau, frozen lima beans, lentils, white beans and chickpeas are among the best sources, followed by liver, duck, blackstrap molasses, fish flour, wheat bran, oysters, dried apricots, walnut and pistachio nuts.

Yet you must consider the amount of iron-rich food normally consumed in determining the amount of iron taken in the diet. For example, while dried apricots are rich in iron, the amount that can be consumed in one meal is comparatively small—as compared with liver or other meat, soybeans, lettuce, lentils or frozen lima beans.

The U.S. RDA for iron is 18 mg.

MAGNESIUM

Sudden infant death, also called crib death, is a tragic and shattering experience. Usually the infant is apparently well nourished and healthy, but a day or two before death may have a mild indefinable complaint for which the physician cannot find a reason. Then, the infant is found dead in his crib. The reason is not known and the tragedy continues to occur.

Dr. Joan L. Cadell put forth a view that sudden infant death is due to magnesium deprivation or deficiency. She confirmed her studies by finding a low magnesium level in the infants who died. Two others, Drs. Swift and Emery, believe that the Cadell theory is well worth further investigation. This becomes especially so because the signs are strikingly similar to the findings when animals die of magnesium deficiency. In animals the signs are just much clearer.

Cadell bases her view on the finding that the infants, usually from a lower economic level, are fed proteins in which calcium and phosphorus are quite high in relation to the magnesium intake. Women in the lower economic strata, when pregnant, consume much more white flour, cabbage, potatoes, dairy foods, white rice, and cannot afford garden-fresh vegetables—hence their magnesium intake is low. They set the stage for the tragedy especially when breastfeeding, since their milk is low in magnesium.

There is a wondrous balance in foodstuff interrelationships: the more calcium and phosphorus that are taken, the less magnesium is absorbed. Conversely, when large amounts of magnesium are given, as intravenously in toxemia of pregnancy, there is a reduction of calcium. In some ways magnesium and calcium, like siblings, have a number of mutual traits, and in others they are antagonistic.

Magnesium is really not a trace mineral or micronutrient because a relatively large amount is present in the body. The daily requirement for an adult is about 400 mg; compare that with copper, which is approximately 2 mg. We are considering it because its importance has long been overlooked and its interest in human nutrition is justifiably increasing. While the need for magnesium in rats has been long recognized, the acceptance that it is a dietary necessity in man was published only in 1957 by Flink and his coworkers and in 1960 by Vallee. Dr. Flink has been deeply engaged in research in magnesium metabolism and Dr. Vallee in micronutrients generally.

Magnesium deprivation can be more serious in a number of other conditions. For example, most vitamins and minerals are at a dangerously low level in alcoholics. But magnesium deficiency especially is said to contribute to brain damage in alcoholics, according to Dr. Stendig-Linberg of the famous Karolinska Institute of Stockholm. His research finds that when there is an adequate magnesium level in alcoholism, the brain damage is much lighter. Others believe that it is the low magnesium level in chronic alcoholics which may precipitate delirium tremens. Drs. McCollister, Flink and Lewis put forth the proposition that the magnesium level is low in alcoholics because alcohol stimulates the excretion of magnesium. There are other troubles due to a low magnesium level; for example, it contributes to the incidence of fractures in children with imperfectly developed bones.

Deficiency of magnesium is manifested by a variety of signs referring to the nervous or muscular systems. They range from muscular irritability or twitching, muscle cramp, muscle spasm (tetany), and weakness to, in severe instances, mental confusion and convulsions.

Depletion of magnesium can occur in malnutrition resulting from restricted diets.

To add to the complexity one cannot easily find magnesium deficiency merely by measuring the level of magnesium in the blood. The most reliable way of testing whether a clinical deficiency does exist is by intravenous injection. Normally 90 percent of the amount should be excreted in the urine within two hours. If 40 percent or more is retained by the body, it is a sign of magnesium deficiency.

Magnesium, in common with many other metals or micronutrients, makes enzymes whole by supplying the metal component. Activating a number of enzyme systems, it supplies the motive power to the all-important adenosine triphosphate (ATP)—the enzyme that makes energy available for all living functions. As ATP is involved in the activity of nerve cells, magnesium becomes largely a nerve micronutrient. We say casually *nerve micronutrient* because a deficiency of magnesium leads to nervous and muscular irritability. But an excess of magnesium can lead to another nervous symptom—depression.

Probably more problems occur due to insufficient magnesium than to its excess. The most likely excess results from injection. While magnesium oxide as well as magnesium sulfate (the latter is epsom salt) can also be taken in excess orally, they merely produce diarrhea.

Magnesium is plentiful in the following foods: seafood, nuts, meats, wheat bran and wheat germ and other whole grains, kelp. It is moderately available in leafy green vegetables, fruits and dairy foods. Its availability or absorption is inhibited in brown or whole wheat bread, oatmeal or any food that contains a good deal of phytic acid, previously mentioned.

The U.S. RDA for magnesium is 400 mg.

MANGANESE

Falling hair is bad. Can falling chest hair be worse? Yes, because chest hair contains three times as much manganese as scalp hair, according to Drs. Rosenstock, Simon and Meyer, psychiatrist and neurologists of Baylor College of Medicine. They were not trying to prevent falling chest hair, but were trying to find out why a man of 22 who was working at a smelting furnace developed severe neurological symptoms. Was it due to manganese poisoning? They didn't know. But since many trace metals or micronutrients are fixed in hair in minute amounts they were trying to find hair where the amounts would be somewhat comfortably larger for measuring. That is how they found the chest-hair link.

Manganese is a migrating micronutrient. For example, there is more than 1,000 times as much manganese in the heart muscle as in blood. But after a heart attack there is a steep decline of the amount of manganese in the heart and a steep rise in the blood.

What is the significance of that? That is not known, but it does suggest that manganese is intimately involved in health and disease.

The pioneer in micronutrients, the same Dr. Schroeder, states that the "evidence that manganese is essential is overwhelming," though deficiency has not yet been found, probably because manganese is so widely distributed in nature. Diets low in manganese are probably due to food refining.

Manganese is one of the micronutrients that can be toxic, exhibiting symptoms of neurological trouble similar to those found in Parkinson's disease. Yet they are reversed by the same remedy as for Parkinson's disease, namely, levo-dopa.

At the first annual Conference on Trace Substances in Environmental Health held in 1967 at the University of Missouri, Dr. George C. Cotzias, who developed the use of levo-dopa in parkinsonism, stated that manganese is most likely an essential micronutrient for man, necessary for bone and tendon metabolism. It is necessary for an enzymatic synthesis of a material called mucopolysaccharide which is deficient in rheumatoid arthritis. Since it is found in many organs in man, it is most probably essential as an enzyme activator. In a number of animals it is definitely found to be essential.

The daily needs in man are estimated to be 5 to 10 mg. Much more can cause a mineral overload and produce liver necrosis.

Manganese is most plentiful in wheat germ, meat, whole buckwheat seed, barley seed, grapenuts (a cereal), pecans, almonds and brazil nuts, dry green split peas, fresh turnip greens, fresh spinach and fresh brussels sprouts.

Do not take manganese supplement unless your doctor recommends it or until we learn more about it.

MOLYBDENUM

We are sure that molybdenum is essential in making railroad tracks. In common with other metals it hardens steel even if used in small amounts. It is also essential in the thriving of many plants and in some animals, as rats and chickens. But its role in man we know virtually nothing about, except a few points that suggest it has a role:

1. It is found in the body of man, especially in skin, liver and kidneys; hence it presumably has a function.
2. It is bound to and involved in the function of certain enzymes.
3. It has an interrelationship with certain other micronutrients in the body, hence presumably serves a function for that reason.

We know that molybdenum is involved with an enzyme related to blood functions but that is not fully understood. No deficiency syndrome has yet been reported.

Its antagonism to an essential micronutrient, namely copper, may shed some light on the function of micronutrients generally in the future. Molybdenum hinders the availability of copper, or it may stimulate its excessive excretions; hence a high molybdenum level may be the same as copper deficiency. This is remedied by the intake of additional copper. Conversely, an increased copper level in the body stimulates the excretions of molybdenum. But such interrelationships among metals do not always work on a tit-for-tat basis.

There are other examples of interrelationships: zinc as well as molybdenum is antagonistic to copper. In some animals a disturbance of reproduction and growth with diarrhea, which was first produced by an excess of zinc and ascribed to zinc and molybdenum deficiency, was actually found to be due to the copper deficiency that these micronutrients produced and not due to toxicity.

Excess molybdenum thus becomes in effect the same as copper deficiency. To deepen the complexity, the function of molybdenum in chickens is inhibited by another micronutrient, tungsten.

Another important function in plants and animals fulfilled by molybdenum is in the body synthesis of sulfur amino acids which are necessary in life.

Do not take supplements of molybdenum unless your doctor recommends them or until we learn more about it.

NICKEL

It was said, not too long ago, that we don't know a nickel's worth about nickel. This may still have been true, except for an event reported in 1970 by Dr. F. W. Sunderman, Jr., of Connecticut University School of Medicine, and somewhat earlier by Drs. D'Alonzo and Pell. It has to do with the high level of nickel that is found in the blood after a heart attack and also after a stroke. It is reasoned that it must have an important role in metabolism if it is involved in such grave conditions.

Why does the nickel level rise so high in the blood after a heart attack? It is not definitely known but it is possibly due to its release from tissues into the blood in response to the metabolic changes in the body produced by a heart attack. It probably has an important role in metabolism by activating certain enzymes or inhibiting others.

No nickel deficiency is known. It is a relatively nontoxic micronutrient found in soils and sea water, and is most plentiful in tea, cocoa, gelatin, red kidney beans.

Do not take nickel supplements; nickel is probably unnecessary as a supplement despite its role, because enough is probably supplied by the common foods.

SELENIUM

One cannot speak of selenium without speaking of vitamin E, as they are intimately related. Selenium is an essential though paradoxical micronutrient. It is toxic, yet has desirable qualities, one of which is inhibiting the oxidation of fats. Its deficiency in animals short-circuits the power packs in the cell called mitochondria. If it is deficient in animals it causes a breakdown in liver function; if in excess it poisons the liver. Some micronutrients, like molybdenum, cobalt, chromium and others, can accentuate the effects of poisoning by selenium, and amazingly, arsenic reduces its poisonous effects. Apparently selenium is necessary and beneficial to man—but not yet is it proved that is so. It does have an intimate relationship to vitamin E, and at times, in some animals, can replace it.

Another paradox: selenium and fluorine are among the highly poisonous micronutrients, yet fluorides reduce caries of teeth, and selenides (derivatives of selenium) poke holes in teeth.

A most interesting observation was made by Dr. Raymond J. Shamberger, from the Cleveland Clinic Foundation, who found, of all things, a relationship between ready-to-eat breakfast cereals and the reduction of stomach cancer. He reported that selenium, in common with other antioxidants such as BHT and BHA which are used to prevent the spoilage of fats and cereals, probably has an anticancer effect which he ascribes to its antioxidant effect.

After this hypothesis occurred to him he found that in cities where selenium is relatively high (in water or vegetation), the rate of stomach cancer is low; and conversely, in cities in which the level of selenium is low, the cancer rate is high. That is how he theorized that the huge increase in use of boxed cereals—which contain the antioxidants vitamin E, BHA or BHT—corresponds to the continuing decline in the incidence of stomach cancer in the United States. Whether that is the reason for the decline of stomach cancer must await further confirmation.

Selenium and Vitamin E

But do not take selenium. It is an extremely poisonous substance. Selenium is related to vitamin E simply because it has *some* of the properties of vitamin E, but it does not have others. About two decades ago it became known that a minute quantity of selenium—one part selenium in *ten million* parts (0.1 ppm) of chicken feed—overcame some of the effects of vitamin E deprivation in chicks.

One of the outstanding researchers on vitamin E, Dr. A. L. Tappel of the University of California at Davis, also reported that the same proportion of selenium—one part in ten million—was able to substitute for vitamin E in some animals, for some conditions. What probably happens is that selenium acts as a fat antioxidant, much the same as vitamin E. But that is not the complete story. Dr. Tappel received the Borden Award from the American Institute of Nutrition in 1973 for his work on the antioxidant effect of vitamin E.

Selenium is extremely toxic for all animals as well as for man. A proportion of only ten parts per million (10 ppm) can kill. Occasionally, pasture lands relatively high in selenium have killed herds of cattle and sheep that have eaten the vegetation.

Selenium is present in probably a smaller quantity in the earth's crust than all but a few elements—only 0.09 part per million, or less than one part in ten million. It is present in sea water in even a smaller amount—about one twentieth as much.

Some of the effects of selenium—but in minute quantities—are similar to those of vitamin E in animals, preventing muscular dystrophy in poults, exudative diatheses in chicks, white muscle disease in cattle and sheep. Some animals probably require selenium even though they may be given vitamin E.

It is fascinating to consider that the role of selenium in preventing liver necrosis in animals was found only when it was realized that selenium was a contaminant in two sulfur-containing amino acids that were administered, methionine and cystine. When these amino acids were purified so that they did not have a trace of selenium, they no longer prevented liver necrosis.

It is not known if selenium is an essential dietary substance in its own right, or if by sparing vitamin E, it potentiates it. One view is that like vitamin E, selenium acts as a free-radical scavenger. It is indeed important in animal feed, but its role in man is uncertain—it is considered essential by some, but not by others.

Minute and varying quantities of selenium occur naturally in seafood (tuna, anchovies, herring, menhaden), brewers' yeast, wheat germ, bran, broccoli, cabbage, tomato, meat and grains. The richest natural sources of selenium are shrimp, lobster, smelt, fish flour, smoked herring fillets, pork kidney, beef kidney and brazil nuts.

Selenium is a highly toxic material. If you take vitamin E do not try to spike it with selenium—it can kill. But there is no objection to eating foods containing selenium as described above, provided that they are not taken in excess in order to build up selenium reserves. They can tear down too.

As you can see there are too many variables—not all of them

understood—to entitle one to be dogmatic about micronutrients.

Do not take selenium as a supplement.

TIN

While tin is one of the metals known since the Bronze Age we know little about its nutritional status today. It may be merely one of the environmental contaminants. It is not toxic except when injected. In fact, much tin must have been taken by people in the early days of the development of canned foods, since cans were then made from tin plate. Today's canned food comes less in contact with tin, since cans are usually lined with an inactive plastic coating.

While tin was at one time used in France as a treatment for boils and acne, that was a pharmacological, not a nutritional use. A comparatively new form with which we now come in contact is in certain toothpastes which contain tin fluoride (stannous fluoride).

Soil is the richest source of tin and probably for that reason fresh vegetables are rich in tin, such as fresh spinach and asparagus, dried split peas and dried navy beans; meat sources are liver, kidney and heart. Part of the tin in our diets possibly may be from canned foods when the plastic coating has ruptured, as in bent cans.

Do not take tin as a supplement.

VANADIUM

Cholesterol is on everyone's lips—and also in the arteries of those who have atherosclerosis. An immense amount of research has been directed to the prevention of stroke and heart attack, believed to be associated with a high cholesterol level in the blood.

As long ago as 1956, Drs. Mountain, Stockel and Stokinger reported that vanadium reduces cholesterol deposition in rabbits. This was followed up three years later by the finding that it can also reduce cholesterol production in man, even in men who have a normal cholesterol level.

Hard-water communities have been found to have a smaller incidence of heart attacks. This has been ascribed to the presence of various micronutrients in the water (see section on magnesium). Vanadium may possibly be the most significant component in hard water contributing to this reported effect.

While vanadium is not yet known as an essential micronutrient for man, it is essential in animals. Dr. Klaus Schwarz, who identified selenium, chromium, tin and other micronutrients in human nutrition, also identified vanadium as essential for growth in animals. He speculates that it will be found essential in man, though no vanadium deficiency in man has been identified. This may well turn out to be the case because it is a common constituent in the body and is excreted in the urine.

It does have functions in the body—namely, as a catalyst for inactivating enzymes that have to do with fat metabolism and certain nerve hormones, called catecholamines. While it can be poisonous, no toxicity has been reported. Vanadium is plentiful in certain foods like seafood, soybeans, corn oil and many vegetables.

Do not take vanadium supplements.

ZINC

Fate deals unkindly with alcoholics. Not only do they fail to take in certain nutrients, including micronutrients, but in addition they void them away in urine at a greater rate than other people. This applies especially though not exclusively to zinc. Excessive losses in urine deplete the body stores of zinc. Many unhappy events can happen in zinc deficiency.

Zinc is recognized as an essential micronutrient for man. Recently it has been found to accelerate wound healing. But it is also necessary in man for growth, sexual maturation, the body syntheses of collagen tissue, in the metabolism of the all-important nucleic acids RNA and DNA, and as a vital component of many enzymes which are the key to a variety of functions in human health.

Some people eat earth—yes, soil. It is called *geophagia*, and is done in some parts of the world, including parts of the South of the United States. In the United States it is based on folklore and has an emotional basis: black pregnant women living in the North often demand earth from their homes in the South to eat here. It may well have an atavistic basis—a desire to be, or have, something close from home to pass on to the child to be born. In eating soil they also pass on something else: a deficiency of certain vital food elements, including micronutrients and especially zinc, because zinc and other micronutrients, while plentiful in the soil, are bound and much less available to the body. Soil also abstracts zinc from the food eaten.

Zinc is not the only micronutrient that suffers by this practice. As with other types of malnutrition, more than one element is usually lacking or deficient, say vitamin A. *Deficiency of zinc makes an existing deficiency of vitamin A worse,* according to Drs. J. C. Smith, Jr., Ellen G. McDaniel and Lois D. McBean of the Washington, D.C., Veterans Administration Hospital and the National Institutes of Health.

A striking example of a similar practice exists in the Middle East, notably in Egypt and Iran, where children suffer severe growth failure to the point of dwarfism. The eating of clay, which is the same as earth-eating, binds both zinc and iron and has produced, especially in boys, an intensely stunted growth and sexual immaturity. Boys of about 17 or 18 are often less than 5 feet tall and their genitals are of the stage of development usually found in boys of 6 years. Malnutrition in other food elements deepens this failure to grow. Supplementation with zinc and iron does help, but does not cancel the effects of the deprivation. That is the reason for Dr. Richard Luecke's (of Michigan State University) recommendation that food sent to underdeveloped nations should be supplemented by zinc to assure growth and sexual maturation.

For other reasons it may also be good to supplement certain foods (such as cereals) with zinc in the United States, because zinc is bound by cereals or other carbohydrate foods. Among other tissues, the male reproductive organs are high in zinc and it probably serves a purpose. This is confirmed by the finding that male reproduction is impaired in zinc deficiency. Other organs rich in zinc are the prostate gland, muscles, kidneys, liver and bone—and eyes. Infants fed by synthetic or artificial diets tend to have a zinc deficiency; this was brought out by Drs. Moynahan and Barnes, who recommended zinc supplementation.

That zinc is vital to animals and that deficiency produces bone deformities, anemia, reproductive dysfunctions among other anomalies, are well-known facts. In many ways, this is mirrored in man. Many enzymes in man have zinc as a component or it activates them. It therefore is not surprising to find that it has recently been found useful therapeutically in certain human dysfunctions.

Precisely how zinc works with enzymes is not known, but it is known that in almost 20 enzyme systems, function is disturbed in zinc deficiency. Hence, the finding that zinc enhances healing of wounds, including leg sores which are ordinarily difficult to heal, is not really surprising. Leg ulcers healed much faster when patients who had a rather low zinc level were given zinc, according to a study by Drs. Hallblood and Lanner. And Dr. Walter J. Pories of the University of Rochester School of Medicine and Dentistry, who has done a great deal of clinical study with zinc in wound healing, confirms these findings.

Drs. Gordon S. Fell, D. P. Cuthbertson, K. Queen and C. Morrison of the Royal Infirmary of Glasgow found that a considerable loss of zinc occurs during stress and the losses can be large with increasing trauma. Surgery is trauma and stress, and they believe that the intake of zinc should be supplemented to make up for such loss, before and during such stresses.

Dr. Robert Henkin of the National Institutes of Health and, independently, Dr. C. M. Hambige of the University of Colorado Medical Center observed another condition that is amenable to zinc supplementation—namely, the loss of the senses of taste and smell, which is called *hypogeusia*. In a substantial proportion of people this condition has responded to treatment by zinc. While these conditions may have another, a serious basis, such as brain tumor, they can and do often develop after a severe common cold or flu. The same loss of taste and often smell at times occurs after surgery (stress) and is associated with a low zinc level in the blood. Zinc has also been described as probably useful in chronic, *noninfected* prostatitis. The reasoning here is not based on stress, but on the premise that supplemental zinc may be especially helpful in reducing symptoms because it supplements zinc in the prostate, which is normally high in zinc. An initial clinical study was done with 15 men suffering from that condition and zinc afforded relief.

Other uses for zinc will most probably be found with increasing research. Some therapeutic findings, however, await confirmation and a good deal of additional study. Among these possible uses for zinc are in atherosclerosis, malabsorption and peripheral vascular disease where circulation in the leg is seriously impeding walking.

But a severe mistake can be made if zinc or any other substance is ballooned out to the proportion of a royal remedy, "good-for-what-ails-you." It can be like the balloon of another trace metal —a lead balloon.

Other conditions may require zinc. For example, Drs. McBean, Smith and Halstead, in their study, found that women during pregnancy and especially those taking oral contraceptives often tend to have low zinc levels. This would suggest that supplementation with zinc would be wise.

Present in virtually all living organisms it would be assumed that zinc has a metabolic role and that there would be up and down levels of zinc when a serious disturbance of health or metabolism is threatened or occurs. The assumption seems to be correct: the zinc level falls in the event of heart attack, kidney disease and pneumonia. In heart attack there is a disturbance in many enzyme levels; and in fact, a confirmatory diagnosis of heart attack is aided by determining the levels in the blood of certain enzymes associated with zinc. Improvement is monitored by repeating those determinations. Also, in cirrhosis of the liver in alcoholism there is a low level of zinc—confirmation of a relationship.

Zinc is chemically similar to cadmium and in fact it is found in nature associated with a minute quantity of cadmium. This is despite the fact that there is an antagonism between cadmium and zinc which can make zinc unavailable and even can poison the zinc-dependent enzymes. (Calcium and phosphorus can also reduce the availability of zinc.) The antagonism is mutual: zinc protects against the effects of cadmium, a toxic metal, which can produce high blood pressure.

Zinc deficiency can occur when the intake is inadequate. But there is another zinc deficiency called *conditional deficiency,* which occurs when a great proportion of the zinc taken in is bound and made unavailable to the body. Such binding, hence conditional deficiency, is produced by cadmium, by vitamin A and, in a lesser proportion, by iron. A deficiency can also be produced by an increased need for zinc, or during stress, which is also a conditional deficiency. Another conditional deficiency is produced by cereals or soybean flour, both containing phytates or phytic acid which binds zinc. (Conditional deficiency occurs in other micronutrients too, and zinc is not unique therein.)

While zinc is not a highly "poisonous" metal, large doses of zinc salts can be toxic. Metal fume fever, for example, is industrial zinc poisoning and occurs upon inhalation of the fumes in smelting operations, where zinc is involved.

Many foods are comparatively rich in zinc, the following containing rich to moderate quantities: seafood, especially oysters, liver, wheat germ and wheat bran, dried green split peas, lima beans, yeast, nuts and milk. While whole grain products are rich in zinc, since they contain phytates they make a portion of it unavailable. Vegetables are not a good source because of variability of zinc content of soil. In fact, Dr. Franck J. Viets, Jr., of the U.S. Department of Agriculture, laments that soils are becoming increasingly deficient in zinc; hence crops growing from such soil will be poor in zinc.

It is well to take zinc supplement. The U.S. RDA is 15 mg.

12

SOME COMMENTS AND INTERPRETATIONS ON MICRONUTRIENTS

SOME GENERALIZATIONS may be made about micronutrients, but bear in mind that they may not apply to every one of them.

Consider the word *poisonous* or *toxic*. Few things are completely nontoxic and, conversely, every material has a toxic potential under certain conditions. For example, if you never think of tomato juice as poisonous or toxic you will probably be correct. But due to its salt content it has a potential for toxicity or harm for the person with high blood pressure who must control his or her salt intake.

When we say that nickel or vanadium is considered nontoxic we should add *by and large*. In fact certain of their salts or derivatives can be and are poisonous. A striking example to demonstrate that point is barium, a metal not known at this time to be of any use to the body. In the form of *barium sulfate,* a totally insoluble salt, it is nontoxic and is used in liberal quantities to make the x-ray cocktails, with the addition of chocolate syrup and water, that you drink before x-rays are taken. The reason is that barium sulfate is opaque to x-rays, and not letting them through, a perfect pattern is made outlining the hollow organ as a stomach or lower bowel, which the barium sulfate coats.

But *barium chloride* is a quick poison causing violent contraction of muscles and arresting heart action. The reason is that it is soluble while the sulfate is not at all soluble. Barium is a poison and solubility makes the difference. When we speak of metals, such as zinc or magnesium, we are usually referring, not to the metal itself, but to a salt or derivative of that metal.

Micronutrients, if taken as supplements, are never taken in the form of the metal but in that of a salt. A salt is a combination of metal and an acid, usually making the metal soluble. And it does make a difference what salt is used. For example, zinc is taken in the form of zinc *sulfate*. But zinc *chloride* is escharotic or caustic.

Certain forms of a metal are more toxic or more irritating than others, or a given form may make the micronutrient unavailable. An example is zinc oxide; in this form the zinc is unavailable because it is largely insoluble.

You cannot say that one micronutrient is more important than another. That would be a sad oversimplification. The body is a finely balanced orchestra wherein each instrument has a task to perform and does so in concert with other instruments. Consider the micronutrients as instruments in this context. Therefore it is a grave error to become fanatic about vitamin C or B_1 or any one micronutrient, because they all have an interrelationship with other micronutrients and other food substances. There can be an ambivalent love-hate relationship. One such example is copper-iron; they have an antagonism under certain conditions. But largely they supplement each other's blood-building function, especially in certain proportions. For example, the body needs 10 times as much iron as copper. If this proportion is disturbed one or both of them can suffer.

Another example wherein a vitamin and micronutrient are involved: in wound healing zinc has been a meritorious discovery. But wound healing is a complex process: both zinc and vitamin C as well as a host of other substances are necessary for the incredibly complex phenomenon of tissue repair to take place.

Here is a partial list of micronutrient interrelationships to illustrate how broad interrelationships can be:

1. Molybdenum blocks the uptake of cobalt and thus interferes with the body synthesis of vitamin B_{12}.
2. Cobalt blocks the uptake of iodine.
3. Molybdenum, in excess, produces copper deficiency.
4. Copper, in excess, increases excretion of molybdenum.
5. Zinc interferes with both copper and iron metabolism.
6. Manganese is better absorbed in iron deficiency, and in fact, iron itself is better utilized in iron deficiency.
7. Zinc and molybdenum are antagonized by copper.
8. Vanadium interferes with iron metabolism and mobilizes iron in the liver.
9. Cadmium depletes zinc.

There are thousands of enzyme systems working in the body and a given micronutrient may inhibit or activate more than one such system. For example, zinc has a role in about 20 such enzyme systems.

It would be logical to assume that a micronutrient has more than one function. That assumption is correct. The following uses or functions of various micronutrients are merely a brief illustration of some important attributes, but this is certainly not a list of all their functions (some are unknown):

Iron—in iron deficiency anemia
Copper—in anemia
Cobalt—in pernicious anemia but active only as part of vitamin B_{12}

Vanadium—lowers cholesterol
Manganese—postulated in rheumatoid arthritis
Chromium—in diabetes to stabilize insulin-sugar metabolism
Fluorine—probably keeps calcium in bones and out of arteries
Zinc—heals wounds
Iodine—guards against thyroid disease

In nutrition, the amounts needed are only estimated for various micronutrients. In certain other conditions, such as diabetes where chromium is involved or in wound healing in which zinc is indicated, a physician should prescribe, since the patient is in no position to diagnose or treat these conditions.

Foods rich in various micronutrients are discussed and listed in their respective sections and form a good basis for their intake. For example, as a general rule only, the following foods are particularly rich in various micronutrients but for specific micronutrients see their appropriate discussions: *seafoods, liver, wheat germ, dry green split peas.*

Should you take supplemental micronutrients in the same sense that vitamins are taken? Yes and no. In the foregoing text dealing with each micronutrient a comment is often made that it would be well to take it. Thus, copper, iodine, iron, magnesium, manganese and zinc are available in the form of mineral tablets.

As for selenium, do not take it as a supplement (see section on selenium), nor vanadium, nor nickel, because too little is known at this time to make an intelligent decision. In the future, it is quite likely that additional study and research on certain other micronutrients, as silicon, for example, may suggest a good reason for taking it as a supplement.

Micronutrients may be useful for more than preventing deficiency. Some investigators believe that they may make the difference between ordinary health and buoyant well-being while aging. Only the future will tell.

You will usually see the micronutrients or other minerals stated in terms of quantities, followed by a phrase such as "as sulfate" or "as oxide" or "as fumarate," etc. What this means, say, in the case of iron, is that the amount of iron fumarate used is equivalent to a given amount of iron. For example, "iron 15 mg as fumarate" means that 45 mg of iron fumarate used is equivalent to 15 mg iron (metal equivalent), as iron fumarate contains 33 percent iron. It is not all iron—if it were it would not be a fumarate, which is a salt of iron.

Similarly, magnesium oxide contains 60 percent magnesium (round figure). Thus, you will need to take 666 mg of magnesium oxide to get 400 mg magnesium (metal equivalent).

Each salt has a different percentage or proportion of its metal. It is not the metal alone that is used in making mineral tablets but the salt.

13

VITAMINS AS SENTINELS

ALL VITAMINS are comparatively newly recognized substances, though they have always existed. The idea that a substance was missing in food, which lack produced a disease, was first proposed in 1913 when it was noted that the growth of rats was inhibited by the absence of a substance in their food. That substance was subsequently called vitamin A—the first one of a family of then new types of nutritional substances.

The whole idea of vitamins was conceptualized by Casimir Funk, who, in fact, originated the name *vitamine*, subsequently modified to *vitamin*. Before his time it was reasoned that the *presence* of a substance which was both foreign and noxious was responsible for the development of certain disease conditions, or that the disease-producing substance may have developed from a natural substance in the body or food that became "spoiled" or poisonous.

Funk's dialectic reasoning suggested that it may well be the *absence* of a desirable element that produced the disease condition. He subsequently proved this in his work on vitamin B_1, or thiamine. But before him, though a deficiency disease—namely, beriberi—had been observed, the cause had not been established as an *absence* of something necessary. Vitamin research took on a much more productive and successful direction after Funk elaborated his hypothesis. This is another example of how conceptualization must first be done before any practical work. A concept is often the light at the end of a tunnel.

Nutrition is not merely a matter of eating enough or of eating to remain well, but more: to function physically and mentally at the optimum—to enjoy buoyant health. Obviously, many other factors in addition to nutrition are involved: there are emotional inputs, societal aspects and economic status, all of which are integrally involved in well-being.

The foregoing deals with nutrition to retain health and well-being. There is also another side to nutrition, one about which we know too little, i.e., nutrition in disease. As long ago as 1958—which is indeed a long time ago in the light of the rapid changes in knowledge that are taking place—Dr. L. E. Holt, Jr., expressed the situation well:

But the future of nutrition as I see it, the big future which is just opening up, is the field of nutrition in disease rather than in health. In the last analysis cells which sicken and die from any pathological process do so because they are improperly nourished. They may die because of failure of some one of the 30-odd essential nutrients that we now recognize. They may die because of an abnormal requirement of one of our presently known nutrients. They may also die for lack of what I may call a conditional nutrient, a nutrient needed only in a particular pathological state, a stress nutrient if you will.

14

ENZYMES: THE SEVEN DWARFS
IN THE CELL ITSELF

To DEFINE ENZYMES in their infinite variety and the roles they play would itself require a number of books. The reason is that in virtually all processes that relate to living organisms or their parts, enzymes are involved—from tanning leather, making buttermilk, getting dough to rise, preserving foods, to breathing and digesting —in fact, in living.

Enzymes are a key, almost *the* key in the sheer process of living, as they are a factor in diagnosis of diseases and their treatment, in the production of food, in growth and maturation. Some enzymes put things together, others take them apart. Enzymes are specific: there is one specific enzyme for each specific task.

This book is not about enzymes, but all living things are related to enzymes. The reason they are briefly considered here is because vitamins and usually micronutrients either activate enzyme systems or inhibit them. For example, thiamine cannot be utilized by the body as such, but as thiamine pyrophosphate it acts as an enzyme. Along the line of its production it needs magnesium to become activated and to spark other enzymes.

What is probably the highest prize on record for a definition was offered by the French government in about 1860. It consisted of a kilo (2.2 lb) of gold and a medal to the person who would adequately define what an enzyme is. While that prize was never claimed, some things have been learned about enzymes in the intervening century.

An enzyme can be roughly defined as a catalyst or middleman, facilitating certain vital functions to take place. Without enzymes most changes in the human organism would not occur, or if they did the changes would be extremely slow. Enzymes are protein molecules, though not all protein molecules are enzymes. They are effective in minute concentrations and often are not used up in a reaction, but they can be worn out, poisoned, as by foreign substances, or killed, as by heat.

For example, the brain is the "biggest customer" of glucose, using it in its metabolism, oxidizing it to carbon dioxide and water. In that process at least a dozen enzymes are involved, each one performing one step. That is what is meant by enzymes being specific—each one has a specific function, only that single function, and none other. Hence, at least a few dozen enzymes may be involved in a single conversion, because such a conversion has many steps.

How are vitamins involved? They act as coenzymes or enzymes.

15

PIGS WITHOUT EYEBALLS:
BIRTH DEFECTS

As LONG AGO AS 1933, a researcher intentionally fed pregnant pigs a diet deficient in vitamin A. They gave birth to some pigs without eyeballs, and their litter mates had other defects. This was a milestone since it was the first demonstration that a deficiency in a nutrient, induced in a pregnant animal, can produce birth defects. The first such nutrient abstracted from the diet was a vitamin, but do not infer from that that vitamin A is a remedy against birth defects.

The causes of birth defects are complex. Generally they can be said to be due to

1. A heritable genetic arrangement that calls forth birth defects under certain conditions.
2. The presence of something that should not be there, such as x-ray treatment, viral infections like German measles or flu, which can produce birth defects in the offspring if the mother is exposed to them during her pregnancy.
3. Certain substances such as thalidomide and several drugs, or excessive amounts of hormones, male, female or others, taken by the mother during pregnancy.

4. A failure to take something, i.e., fasting, or deficiency in a nutrient that is necessary in the development and maturation of the fetus. While these are usually the same nutrients that are necessary for good health for the mother—pregnant or not—there is an accentuated need for certain vitamins and minerals in pregnancy.

That this problem needs more study is clear in view of the general lack of predictability and the tragedy that a defective child represents. Even if a child is not defective it may not develop to its proper potential if the mother is not optimally nourished during and even before her pregnancy. In fact, Dr. Myron Winick, director of the Institute of Human Nutrition of Columbia University, emphasizes that "undernutrition of the mother may permanently reduce the number of brain cells in her offspring."

Malnutrition—this applies to all nutrients and is not limited to vitamins and micronutrients—during brain growth may produce lasting mental deficits. A period of rapid brain growth is approximately five months before birth to about the end of the first year of life.

Dr. Delbert H. Dayton of the National Institute of Child Health and Development (of the National Institutes of Health) divides brain growth in animals, and presumably in humans, into three phases:

1. A period during which the cells increase in *number*
2. A period during which they increase both in *number* and in *size*
3. A period during which the cells increase in *size*

Malnutrition during the first and second periods hinders the development of cell size, presumably with permanent damage.

It should not be inferred that the nutritional aspect of brain development is the whole picture. *Lack of emotional input is a form of deprivation—a sort of emotional malnutrition.*

Dr. Sohan L. Manocha, associate professor of neurohisto-chemistry at Emory University, also clearly confirms that the peak period of brain growth takes place prenatally, does not cease until after the first year, and that mothers' who are substantially mal-nourished bring forth offspring who have a reduced number of cells. The flippant phrase "your brain didn't grow" may be a tragic reality. *The mother programs the future of her baby.* Malnutrition in babies is expressed not only in physical but also in mental deficits as they grow.

Dr. Manocha wisely points out that the *young female* is the crucial nexus in this state of affairs, because it is the nutritional education of the mother that will have a lasting effect on her babies. But nutritional knowledge often fights vainly against cultural influences which include the highly complex social, economic, religious and cultural realities. Politicians tell us what an affluent country this is, and how astronomical our standard of living. But a poor economic environment precludes the many advantages of our society, even nutritional education of the mother. Bear in mind that about three fourths of people at the lower economic level do not get newspapers. About 90 percent do not know what to buy for want of basic information.

We need honesty and empathy to overcome this widespread problem. Nutritional knowledge alone, which is often hawked as the redemption for all things that ail one, is not enough. Man in the affluent society has even lost the instinctive knowledge that animals have for food for their well-being.

Pregnancy is a time of immense upheaval. Among other changes, and many of them for the worse, anemia in pregnancy is more frequent than is often believed, according to Dr. Jane Desforges of the hematology laboratory at Tufts University. In

spite of her belief that a normal pregnancy does not require supplementation with extra iron, she avers that there is often a
hidden iron depletion in the mother for a number of reasons,
among which are numbered previous hemorrhages, excessive
menstrual bleeding, and the continuing need for iron for growth
in the case of pregnant teenagers.

Another major need in pregnancy for the mother, as well as
for the fetus, Dr. Desforges reminds us, is for folic acid or folacin,
which may be required for a number of factors aside from pregnancy. These other factors can include taking drugs which, while
necessary, may interfere with the utilization of the vitamins she
may be getting; other complications that increase the need for
vitamins are pregnancy vomiting, diarrhea or the mother's alcoholism.

Specializing in blood research, Dr. Desforges emphatically
urges pregnant women to undergo a comprehensive blood study
to uncover any needs that they may have which can be satisfied
to their benefit as well as that of the fetus.

What are the vitamin deficiencies that produce birth defects in
animals and many in man? Vitamins A, C, D, E, B_2, pantothenic
acid, B_{12}, niacin, folic acid and probably others as well. Articles in
newspapers often warn against the possibility of birth defects
from the use of vitamins. If there is a uniform danger to pregnant
women it is from undernutrition, not from vitamins.

An official statement on the relation of excess vitamins to pregnancy is the following paragraph from the Report on Maternal
Malnutrition of the American College of Obstetricians and Gyne-
cologists:

While available evidence does not indicate vitamin supplements have a beneficial effect, neither does it generally
suggest harmful sequelae. A possible exception, however, is
vitamin D. Some evidence suggests—though by no means

does it prove—a relationship between maternal hypervita-
minosis D and the subsequent development of severe infan-
tile hypercalcemia with craniofacial abnormalities and
supravalvular aortic and pulmonic stenosis. For this reason no
increase in vitamin D intake is advised during pregnancy. It
should be pointed out that the recommended daily intake of
vitamin D (400 IU, pregnant or not) is the amount contained
in 1 quart of vitamin D-enriched milk.

What this means is simple. Don't take more vitamin D anyway.

Birth defects can occur from a deficiency of folic acid or
through taking an antagonist to folic acid (see chapter 18 on antivitamins) which prevents its utilization. That amounts to folic
acid deprivation.

Can micronutrients prevent birth defects? New and intensely
interesting findings were reported by Dr. Lucille S. Hurley, professor of nutrition at the University of California at Davis, who
prevented birth defects in rats by supplementing the diets of pregnant rats with manganese. Certain strains of rats and mice are
known to develop birth defects, one of which is a loss of muscular
coordination (ataxia). These animals are bred for that purpose
in order to have a model on which genetic defects can be studied
and remedied and hopefully applied to man.

At the second annual Conference on Trace Substances held
at the University of Missouri in 1968, Hurley reported that she
gave supplementary manganese in the diet to a group of pregnant rats of the strain that develops these birth defects. Another
group of rats, of the same strain, received the identical diet but
without the manganese supplement. The following extraordinary
things happened:

1. The offspring of the rats that received the manganese supplement did not develop ataxia.

2. The offspring of the group that did not receive manganese did develop ataxia.

3. When the offspring of the first group of rats that did not develop ataxia was subsequently bred without manganese supplement, it gave birth to litters that *did* have the genetically transmitted birth defect—ataxia.

This means that while manganese does not change the genes (because the offspring of the offspring of the first group of rats developed ataxia), manganese supplements do suppress or inhibit the manifestations of the birth defect in rats that carry the hereditary strain of a birth defect.

Dr. Hurley had a similar experience in prevention of birth defects even more quickly, by the use of other micronutrients, namely zinc and magnesium. Deprivation of these also causes failure of fetal development, i.e., birth defects.

While this applies to animals, it may well also apply to man. Drs. Lyndon A. Peer, Harry W. Gordon and William G. Bernhard pointed out that the fact that birth defects can be induced in animals offers hope that they can probably be prevented in man. Their own experience at St. Barnabas Medical Center with 400 human pregnancies which resulted in offspring with birth defects is striking. Of the 400 women, 306 had not had birth defects in their families before. But 275 women of the 306 had not taken vitamin supplements during early pregnancy or before. Despite that fact one cannot jump to a conclusion and immediately ascribe the birth defects to be due to vitamin deprivation, as these people may possibly have had an adequate intake of vitamins from their diet. Nonetheless, the relationship between the high incidence of birth defects and failure to take vitamin supplements is so highly suggestive that Dr. Peer and his associates recommend an intake of vitamin supplements not only at the first suspicion of pregnancy but also to prospective brides, since they may become pregnant shortly after marriage.

Knowledge on what produces and what may prevent birth defects in humans is extremely sparse. Much more is known about animals. The reason is because one can experiment on animals—feed them intentionally a deficient diet which can produce birth defects, then vary the diet to determine what can prevent them. The National Foundation is devoted to the study of birth defects, and through its funding some knowledge has been developed. Yet, at its convention in New York in the spring of 1973, no paper was presented which clearly outlined what deficiencies are inimical to normal births.

The expression *birth defects* is used in this chapter. You will meet other terms, such as congenital abnormalities, congenital deformities, or genetically induced birth abnormalities. These terms are all synonymous. You will also meet the term *teratology* in this connection. Teratology is the study of birth defects; a teratogen is an agent that induces them (like thalidomide); teratogenic is an adjective describing a substance or condition that induces birth defects, such as x-rays.

A genetically induced condition like birth defect is controlled by genes and chromosomes. People often assume that they are synonyms. Chromosomes and genes are *not* the same—they are different substances. Chromosomes are fine, less-than-hairlike strands in the nucleus of a cell. (Cell nuclei can be seen only with a microscope, which will give an idea of the infinitesimal size of chromosomes.) Genes are yet smaller structures found *in* the chromosomes. Genes determine the traits carried from generation to generation, predestining individual traits. In that fashion they direct the manifestations of heredity. The genes are probably composed of nucleic acid, namely deoxyribonucleic acid, commonly referred to as DNA. DNA acts as a pattern or template from which another nucleic acid, ribonucleic acid, commonly referred to as RNA, carries the genetic message to replicate the traits of a species. This is the currently accepted theory; it may well be modified as our knowledge in this area continues to increase.

16

THE BIG MINERALS: CALCIUM, PHOSPHORUS, POTASSIUM AND SODIUM

WHILE EMPHASIS in this book is put on the micronutrients, i.e., the trace minerals, there are also other important minerals not called trace minerals because more than traces of them are necessary for the body to function. Unlike trace minerals or micronutrients, people are more familiar with them.

However, brief summaries of the role of each of those important minerals (also called *macro*minerals)—calcium, phosphorus, sodium and potassium—are given here for the frame of reference they may supply and because they are also mentioned in other places in this book.

The RDA for calcium and phosphorus varies with age and other conditions such as pregnancy. Therefore, see chart on the inside front cover for full details. The U.S. RDA is inside the back cover.

CALCIUM AND PHOSPHORUS

You cannot talk of calcium unless you also talk of phosphorus because they are interdependent—another example of the interrelationship of minerals and even other nutrients. One reason for their interdependence is based on the endocrine system: the utilization of calcium and phosphorus depends on the function of certain endocrine glands, as the parathyroid gland.

Calcium and phosphorus are necessary for the formation of bones and teeth, a reason why pregnant women need more calcium and phosphorus than other adults. Mothers who are breast-feeding need extra calcium for enhancing the quality of the milk they produce and to overcome the calcium drains of lactation.

Adults ordinarily need no supplementary calcium and phosphorus but that in food except the amounts needed to balance the output and input. If the output from the body of each is greater than the input, the body is said to be in negative calcium or phosphorus balance, and each must be taken from other tissues; in such a case, supplementation is desired.

Calcium and phosphorus are available in food, which usually will be sufficient for ordinary but not for therapeutic use. See the table later on calcium and phosphorus in foods to get an idea of their relative content. It is believed by some that older people need more calcium as a daily quota, in order to make up for that lost through osteoporosis, which is a thinning of the density of bone through loss of calcium. But whether the extra amount is utilized is not certain.

Calcium and phosphorus are also necessary for the adequate function of the nervous system but for different reasons: calcium to allow the normal transmission of signals in the nervous system, and phosphorus to make a component of the energy enzyme called ATP, previously mentioned under the B vitamins.

Another need for calcium is for proper blood clotting. The needs for phosphorus include those for the metabolism of certain carbohydrates. Excess amounts taken are excreted largely in the feces, also in the urine. The proportionate needs of calcium and

Calcium and Phosphorus Content of Selected Foods. Expressed as mg per 100 gm of Edible Portion (Figures Rounded Off)

	Calcium	Phosphorus
Beans: Common, mature seeds, dry		
White, raw	150	425
White, cooked	50	150
Black, brown or bayou, raw	135	420
Lima: immature, raw	50	140
immature, cooked	45	120
mature, dry, raw	70	380
mature, dry, cooked	30	150
Mung, mature, dry, raw	120	340
Beef, estimated average	10	150
Brazil nuts	190	700
Bread, white, estimated average	75	90
Cornmeal	5	100
Grapefruit	20	20
Kale	225	60
Oatmeal	55	400
Peanuts	75	400
Peanut butter	75	400
Potatoes, white	10	55
Potatoes, sweet	30	50
Salmon, canned, pink	190	290
Sardines, estimated average	400	600
Tuna, canned, solids	10	350

phosphorus are ideally even, i.e., 1:1. Some authorities believe that the proper calcium-phosphorus ratio should be 1:1.5, i.e., one and a half times as much phosphorus as calcium.

The question always arises whether large quantities (1) will be absorbed or (2) can be harmful. The body metabolism for these minerals is such that excessive quantities are usually not absorbed, but they can be harmful if, for example, calcium is taken with a large quantity of vitamin D, which hugely increases the absorption of calcium and may lead to calcification (a calcium deposit in the tissues). Also, as it can be retained in case of kidney malfunction, excessive phosphorus can become toxic.

Some conditions, however, can inhibit adequate absorption. One is malabsorption, which inhibits absorption of calcium. Another example is the ingestion of aluminum hydroxide gel for stomach ulcer, which markedly reduces the absorption of phosphorus because it forms an insoluble complex with it, which is excreted. Also, certain foods, such as cereals, can bind calcium and thus hinder its absorption.

The U.S. RDA for calcium is 1 gm. The U.S. RDA for phosphorus is 1 gm. For RDA see inside front cover.

SODIUM AND POTASSIUM

You will probably never be deficient in sodium or potassium under normal circumstances even if your diet is less than optimum. But you may want to know some aspects of the function of these twins, which work together as well as antagonistically, because there are conditions that may require an extra intake.

You cannot normally take an excessive amount of sodium or potassium in your food, unless you coat your food white with salt, or unless you have high blood pressure or a kidney condition. In these latter cases you should restrict your intake of sodium and potassium.

But both sodium and potassium are necessary in your diet. They are needed in metabolism of the cells and the function of the events that take place between the cells. They also have a role in the distribution and utilization of water in the tissues. (See Chaper 17 on water.)

If you lose an inordinate amount of sodium, as in excessive

perspiration, you should replace not only the water lost but also the sodium. You can do that by taking salt tablets, in moderation, with the water. Recent work has also disclosed that the replacement of potassium is as important. However, while you can take salt tablets to replace the sodium (though an occasional report says that it is not necessary), do not take tablets to replace potassium but instead use one of the potassium-rich foods you will find in the table at the end of this section.

Replacement of sodium and potassium may also be necessary after severe diarrhea or vomiting, on which supplementation your doctor will advise you; he may also wish to supplement other minerals, as magnesium, calcium or phosphorus. Salt is also necessary in pregnancy, though at times it should be restricted in the event of accumulation of water, as in edema, or in high blood pressure during pregnancy.

While sodium is the principal salt *outside* the cell, potassium is the chief salt *inside* the cell. Yet they work in concert, going through cell membranes to assure equilibrium of various functions.

Sodium is needed for the various functions of the nervous system. When we speak of sodium we usually mean table salt—the form in which we obtain most of the sodium in our bodies.

The intake of sodium is usually restricted in high blood pressure. While sodium probably does not produce high blood pressure, it may accentuate it or a tendency to it, though some authorities believe that sodium is actually involved in its development. But even people with high blood pressure need some sodium, in small amounts, which is available in most foods.

The so-called American diet—varied though it is—is estimated to contain from 6 to 15 gm salt daily. All that is normally needed per day is about .05 to 1 gm. Therefore, do not ordinarily take sodium supplements.

Potassium is needed for the proper functioning of a number of systems of the body, including the nervous and muscular tissues, for the buildup of protein, and as an ingredient in producing the reserve energy that is conferred by muscle sugar (glycogen).

There is normally no potassium deficiency, and you need no potassium supplements in addition to that you take in normal foods. When you need a potassium supplement, your doctor will prescribe it.

As with sodium, potassium is found in most foods. If too much is taken it is excreted provided that you have a sound kidney system. But potassium can be built up in the body and be retained in case of kidney or heart disease. More frequently, there is a loss of potassium in certain conditions. For example, chronic alcoholics, who have so many other deficiencies, often may also be deficient in potassium. During fasting or dieting there is a loss of potassium as well as in diarrhea, in vomiting or when taking diuretics or cortisonelike drugs.

When there is a potassium loss there may be muscle weakness, cramps, diarrhea or vomiting produced by the low potassium, in addition to loss of appetite, apathy and listlessness. Either too little or too much potassium in the body can produce such grave signs as evidence of heart disease on the electrocardiogram by interfering with the electrical conductivity of the heart muscle. In fact, a low level of potassium may interfere with the effect of digitalis given for heart disease, making the effect stronger and possibly precipitating toxicity.

Do not take potassium as a supplement unless your doctor recommends it.

Following is a table of foods, commonly used, which contain sodium and potassium, selected with an eye for foods rich in potassium; sodium is much more easy to come by. The quantities of foods chosen are those that are commonly sufficient for a meal.

Hence, the list does not contain foods that, while rich in potassium, as horseradish, are consumed merely in very small quantities as condiments or flavors. Similarly, while frozen concentrates of orange juice are extremely rich in potassium, they are not listed because they are not consumed in that form. However, orange juice and tomato juice in ready-to-drink form, whether made from concentrate or fresh, are listed in the table.

The sodium and potassium contents of certain foods, such as potatoes or beans, are given in both raw and cooked forms. While you do not eat raw potatoes, do be aware what salts are thrown out with the cooking water. All figures given are rounded off.

Sodium and Potassium Content of Selected Foods Relatively High in Potassium. Expressed as mg per 100 gm of Edible Portion (*Figures Rounded Off*)

	Sodium	Potassium
Almonds: dried	4	775
roasted, salted	200	775
Apples: raw	1	110
butter	2	250
Apricots: raw	1	280
dehydrated, uncooked	1,260	14,000
Baby foods, high protein with added nutrient	650	1,000
Bananas: raw, yellow or red	1	370
dehydrated	4	1,500
Beans: common, mature seeds, dry		
white, raw	20	1,200
white, cooked	7	400
black, brown, bayou, raw	25	1,040
lima: immature, raw	2	650
immature, cooked	1	420
mature, dry, raw	4	1,500
mature, dry, cooked	2	600
mung, mature, dry, raw	6	1,030

	Sodium	Potassium
Beef, estimated average	60	370
Bran, added sugar & malt extra	1,060	1,070
Brazil nuts	1	700
Bread: white enriched	500	85
whole wheat	525	275
Broccoli, raw spears	15	380
Buckwheat, whole grain	—	450
Carrots, raw	45	340
Cocoa: dry powder, estimated average high-fat or breakfast cocoa, *plain*	6	1,500
processed with alkali (which is the common form of soluble cocoa)	717	650
Coffee: instant, dry powder	72	3,250
beverage	1	36
Cow peas, including blackeye peas, mature seeds, dry, raw	35	1,025
Eggs, whole, fresh or frozen	122	129
Grapefruit, raw (all kinds, estimated average)	1	150
Halibut, raw	55	450
Milk: cow's whole or skim, average	50	140
dry, whole	400	1,300
skim (nonfat solids)	530	1,745
Orange juice, raw or canned	1	200
Peanuts, raw or roasted, unsalted	5	675
Pears	2	130
Peas: mature seeds, dry, whole, raw	35	1,000
without seed coat, raw	40	900
cooked	13	300
Pineapple juice, canned, unsweetened	1	150
Pork, cooked, estimated average	65	300
Potatoes: raw	3	400
baked in skin	4	500
boiled in skin	3	400
boiled after paring	2	285
Potato chips (up to)	1,000	1,500

	Sodium	Potassium
Rice: brown, raw	10	215
brown, cooked	282	70
white, raw	5	90
white, cooked	375	28
Rolls, commercial:		
hard or plain rolls	625	100
Danish pastry	366	110
Salmon, canned, solids & liquid		
no added salt	50	400
Salt, ordinary table		
(listed for comparison)	38,760	4
Sardines, Atlantic, canned in oil:		
solids and liquid	510	560
drained solids	820	590
Sardines, Pacific, canned in brine:		
solids and liquid	760	260
Seaweed: kelp	3,000	5,275
Shrimp	190	230
Soybean flours, high or low fat, estimated average	1	1,750
Squash, all varieties, estimated average	1	300
Tomato juice, canned: regular	200	225
dietetic	3	225
Wheat bran, crude, comm. milled	9	1,120
Wheat germ, crude, comm. milled	3	825
Yeast: brewers', debittered	120	1,900
torula	15	2,000

(Food tables in this book are derived from the standard Composition of Foods, Agriculture Handbook No. 8, U.S. Department of Agriculture, 1968. Expressed in terms of milligrams per 100 grams edible portion of food as customarily consumed. The amount of 100 gm is equivalent to about 3½ oz.)

17

WATER

Aquatic animals live with water all around them. We have a sea of water inside of us, without which nothing could function. Water is the most important dietary constant, if there were such a thing as the *one* most important thing in nutrition. We can do without almost any nutrient for a short time but not without water. Water is not a vitamin, nor mineral, nor micronutrient—it is not a nutrient at all—but it is imperative for our functioning because all substances act in an environment of water. In fact, except for fat and bones, the human body is three-fourths water.

Water, the solvent in which all events and interactions take place, is the vehicle for (1) the transport and utilization of nutrients, (2) the discharge of excrements, (3) cooling the body through perspiration and (4) the circulation of the blood, in which water is the vehicle.

We need about five pints of water daily—more if the water output is excessive, as through perspiration, or if the urinary output is greater than normal, as in diabetes. Infants are most sensitive to water deprivation, either through sweating or more particularly through diarrhea or vomiting. They may become dried up—dehydrated—more easily than adults. In an infant this can be life-threatening.

Attention to the water intake is also necessary in older people with their reduced functions, such as elimination. While many such people cannot take large amounts of water owing to heart or kidney dysfunctions, they do need a smaller but regular input. Water can be made more palatable to some by flavorings, such as small additions of lemon or grape juice. Skim milk, further diluted half and half with water and flavors, may be more easily taken.

Everyone needs water. Do not use milk or coffee as a substitute for water for you will build up other substances such as fat and calcium in milk, caffeine in coffee or sugar in soft beverages which you can do better without. This does not mean that you should drink water instead of milk or coffee; but the reverse is equally injudicious.

We expel water in forms other than perspiration and urination: breathing, which is done continuously during life, disposes of a substantial amount of water vapor in the expired air.

Water is utilized in different ways in the body. Sodium and potassium are the principal salts that control its accumulation, distribution, retention and discharge. The glandular system is also a controlling factor, such as the pituitary and adrenal glands, which control diuresis and also elaborate an antidiuretic hormone. In addition, the kidneys function as a checkpoint: how much to allow for discharge or for absorption and recirculation.

The following figures will give you an idea of the ubiquity and enormity of the role of water—how much is used by each system daily.

	Pints daily
Saliva	1 to 3
Stomach juices	3 to 5
Intestinal juices	3 to 8
Perspiration	1 to 8

While water is everywhere in our bodies, we can drown in a teacupful—if it is inhaled or if it accumulates in the lungs.

18

ANTIVITAMINS AND VITAMIN TOXICITIES

VITAMINS HAVE SOME close personal enemies—the antivitamins. Antivitamins work against vitamins by blocking their desirable actions. And some vitamins can be toxic themselves under certain conditions:

1. Vitamins A and D can be toxic in very large doses.
2. Under specific blood conditions, vitamin K can become toxic.
3. They may occasionally, though rarely, produce an allergic reaction, especially applicable to injections of B_1.

Let us look on these little-known facets of the vitamins and some micronutrients.

Antivitamins or the "Trojan Horse Syndrome"

An antivitamin is a substance that is often chemically so similar to a vitamin that the tissues get fooled and accept it. When a tissue metaphorically bites into an antivitamin it breaks its own metaphoric teeth. In fact, that is the reason the substance is an antivitamin: it can "fool" the tissue up to a point but at that point it comes out of its Trojan Horse—it prevents the uptake or availability of the genuine vitamin. Antivitamins can also be described as antimetabolites, since they throw the proverbial monkey-wrench into the metabolic machinery. There are several ways in which the antivitamins or antimetabolites work their undesirable effect:

1. They can compete with a vitamin for a tissue to accept them, which tissue thus becomes deprived of the vitamin it has lost in the competition.
2. They can inhibit or completely stop a vital enzyme reaction in which a vitamin takes part.
3. They can otherwise clog a system to prevent utilization of the vitamin they have replaced.

Do not be concerned that you will get an antivitamin in your food—that is rare and happens only in certain toxic foods. It's easier to pick up athlete's foot. Antivitamins, however, are useful for another purpose: in animal nutrition they can produce a severe vitamin deficiency so that one can find out what happens in that deficiency. However, some drugs act as antivitamins or antimetabolites. They are not used intentionally for that purpose but for another condition.

Many vitamins have their antivitamins and some have more than one. For example, thiaminase is an antivitamin to thiamine, or vitamin B_1. This is a minor or moderate problem in Japan where raw fish is eaten. Thiaminase is found in raw fish and can kill an animal that has eaten it. Don't eat raw fish (this does not apply to uncooked but otherwise processed fish such as smoked or pickled herring).

There are other antivitamins to thiamine: deoxypyrithiamine, oxythiamine and pyrithiamine. They prevent the formation of a phosphate coenzyme in which form thiamine is utilized. Fortunately, the competition between thiamine and its antivitamins can be reversed, as a substantially increased amount of thiamine successfully competes with the competitor and overcomes it. Nothing succeeds like excess, according to Oscar Wilde.

Other vitamins and their antagonists or antivitamins are as follows:

Riboflavin (B_2) antivitamins:	isoriboflavin; galactoflavin
Pyridoxine (B_6) antivitamins:	deoxypyridoxine (isoniazid, a drug used in the treatment of tuberculosis, also has an antagonistic effect on vitamin B_6)
Niacin antivitamin:	3-acetylpyridine; pyridine-3-sulfonic acid
Pantothenic acid antivitamin:	omega-methylpantothenic acid
Biotin antivitamin:	raw egg white, which contains a substance called avidin
Folid acid antivitamin:	methotrexate or aminopterin, used as a drug in the treatment of other conditions, as cancer
Vitamin K antivitamin:	dicoumarol, which is really not an antivitamin but an antimetabolite— a small but often substantial difference

Not all antimetabolites are antivitamins, but all antivitamins are antimetabolites. Note the similarity in name between some vitamins and their antivitimins; just because of the similarity in structure they can act as antivitamins.

What are important, however, are the drug-induced vitamin deficiencies. When you take a drug that happens to have an antivitamin effect, you may develop a vitamin deficiency. Dr Daphne A. Roe, associate professor of nutrition of Cornell University, has recently summarized some data on drug-vitamin interaction. Among examples are folic acid deficiency or vitamin D deficiency induced by anticonvulsant drugs, taken by people to control epilepsy, or deficiency of vitamin C and folic acid in women who take oral contraceptives. A similar deficiency can be produced in people who take antidiabetic drugs. A deficiency of pyridoxine or niacin may result from intake of an antituberculosis drug, isonicotinic acid hydrazide; or there may be a vitamin K deficiency in people who are taking anticoagulants in the treatment of thrombophlebitis or as a protective against a second heart attack.

Toxicity

Some vitamins can be toxic, chiefly vitamins A and D, if taken in very large doses for a considerable length of time; vitamin K if taken for a shorter time.

Vitamin A intoxication is occasionally reported, especially with massive intake over a long period of time, such as 25,000 IU daily for infants and 100,000 IU daily or more for adults. Its toxicity may manifest itself in various degrees of such skin symptoms as sores or swelling, in bone or joint pain, or in nervous or muscular symptoms. The toxic reports may possibly be overstated, as people who eat liver frequently consume large quantities of vitamin A. Beef liver contains about 60,000 IU vitamin A per 4-oz portion; polar bear liver, incidentally, is about 10 times richer in vitamin A than beef liver.

A more serious state is vitamin D toxicity. It raises calcium in tissues to a serious level and may cause calcification of soft tissues, thus affecting the kidneys and producing gastrointestinal symptoms, kidney stones or kidney failure, high blood pressure, even mental retardation, and it was recently reported to produce a rise in the cholesterol level of the blood.

Another effect—though not an unexpected one, due to the calcification that can occur in vitamin D poisoning—is the acceleration of the signs of age. Aging is associated with generalized degeneration of tissues and functions. Hence, the toxic effect of a substance that accelerates the signs of aging probably has an effect that is more broad than expected.

Vitamin K is a necessary vitamin. But according to Dr. W. A. Cochrane, quoted in the *Medical Letter,* in pregnancy near term it can produce a type of jaundice in the newborn which can lead to a neurological degeneration called kernicterus. The *Letter* mentions a report made in 1965 which in turn quotes work done in the 1950's. Little if anything was reported in the interim.

Specific situations have been occasionally reported wherein otherwise salubrious vitamins can actually produce a deficiency. Such a situation arises when a larger amount of vitamins given is suddenly withdrawn, at which time the body cannot accustom itself to the absence of vitamins. This, as quoted in a singular case by Dr. Gordonoff, may possibly be more true of water-soluble vitamins, which are not stored in the body, but probably is not applicable to fat-soluble vitamins, most of which are stored.

A similar situation described by Dr. Cochrane is the use of large quantities of water-soluble vitamins during pregnancy. After birth the infant may develop scurvy when withdrawn from the vitamin C–rich environment of the mother, or similarly may develop convulsions when it leaves the pyridoxine-rich environment of the mother. These probabilities have been postulated and implied by Cochrane but are not otherwise found in the literature.

Allergic skin reactions have been rarely reported from the following vitamins: B_1, B_{12} and nicotinic acid. The incidence is negligible.

Some micronutrients can be toxic. Specific mention has been made in each section pertaining to the individual micronutrient where it applies. Some are clearly toxic, such as selenium. In other micronutrients toxicity or disturbance can be produced by overload, as in the case of copper or iron, which may call forth specific symptoms or interfere with the utilization of other micronutrients.

There is an increasing consumption of soybeans or soybean flour. Nutritionally, soybeans are a fine source of protein. However, they inhibit the growth of animals and can also block the utilization of certain micronutrients unless the soybeans have previously been heated. Heat destroys the interfering enzyme.

Naturally, neither soybeans nor any other dried beans are eaten raw. Normal cooking destroys the inhibiting enzyme they contain. The reason for the paragraph above is to caution the user to avoid fanatic recipes which recommend making a drink consisting of soybean flour, yeast, milk, etc., mixed in a blender. Soybean flour is fine for baking—but not for eating raw.

19

OBESITY*

Definitions

Obesity is an increase of body weight, predominantly fat, usually 10 percent or more above what a "normal" weight is considered to be according to the standard height-frame-weight tables. Obesity is always overweight, though overweight is not necessarily obesity. Overweight is an increase of 10 percent or more of body weight (not necessarily fat) over that considered to be the normal weight by these tables. While overweight and obesity are not necessarily synonyms, they can well be considered to be the same for practical purposes.

Hunger is a painful or at least an uncomfortable sensation in the stomach. It occurs usually when the stomach is empty. Hunger is accompanied by peristaltic waves in the stomach walls, felt as or accompanied by pangs ("hunger pangs") or a hollow feeling, crying to be filled. It is relieved by food intake—though not invariably, as will be discussed later.

Appetite is something else; it is a pleasant anticipatory feeling characterized by a desire for the pleasant sensation of eating.

* This chapter is taken from the author's previous book, *Without Prescription,* Simon and Schuster, publishers, copyright © 1972 by Erwin Di Cyan.

Cause

There is one simple cause for obesity: the consumption of more food than is necessary for outgoing energy expenditure. This applies even in the rare occasion when obesity is due to a "glandular" condition or due to a genetic predisposition. In those conditions, too, the energy expenditure is also less than the food intake. Either energy expenditure is too low or food intake is too high. There may be a number of reasons why certain persons have a smaller output of energy, not balanced with the intake of food.

Discussion and Cautions

It is often a mistake to urge people to reduce. Fat serves a purpose. The process of acquiring it is associated with the comfort of eating—usually too well. Food has a sedative action; the relaxation and unwinding after having dined or supped are traditional. Fat or obesity is also a buffer. Metaphorically, it protects the fat person from the outside world—warding off anxiety, exorcising the devils figuratively that literally do not exist. But even if they exist only symbolically or figuratively, they appear real!

Food is a comfort, an anxiety-reducing measure due to its sedative or relaxing value. The greater the anxiety the greater or more frequent will be the intake of food, in the search for equanimity, peace, relaxation, or to do battle with the frustrations that create anxiety. And the greater or more frequent the intake of food, the more it adds to body weight, hence obesity.

But something bizarre happens: the abnormally high intake of food with the intention, conscious or otherwise, of reducing anxiety and perhaps enhancing acceptance by the outside world has just the opposite effect. It increases the probability of rejections, due plainly to an ungainly appearance.

The traditional example of the fat girl is well known: she does not have a satisfactory social life, and spends her evenings home because few people ask for her company. She stays home—and eats candy—becomes fatter—decreases her chances for social relations—therewith eats more—further decreasing her opportunities.

The chain of evidence leading to the causes of obesity is primarily psychological. Most people overeat for psychological reasons. There is a way to correct obesity, but it is best to prevent it. The correction of obesity rests on two pillars, (1) caloric restriction and (2) psychological reevaluation. Both must be present to reduce weight and, above all, to keep it reduced. We shall discuss the details later.

While it is said that fat people do not want to reduce, consciously or not, they cannot or should not be blamed or condemned for their obesity, as fat does serve an inner psychological need. Successful weight reduction is obtained by the reevaluation of the psychological need served by fat or by the process of its acquisition. Restriction of caloric intake without a more basic insight into the reason for caloric overacquisition will not have lasting benefits, because the obese person on a weight-reducing diet will not stick to it long.

Another difficulty found with weight reduction is based on the fact that food is also a cultural phenomenon. The dinner or feast as a cultural or religious event is well known. It is considered socially gauche to refuse to partake of food orgies, which many festive occasions represent. In the family matrix, the same cultural or social phenomenon takes place when a family celebrates an event.

In addition, there come into play the psychodynamics of family interaction. For example, a mother will frequently urge, implore, scream, in her attempts to push food into her children. Her basic reason is not nutritional concern. She may not be aware that she is not a loving mother. She stuffs her children with food to substitute for the love that she cannot give them—because she may not have it. A seductive or manipulative mother also uses food, among other devices, to gain her ends. The foundation for obesity is thus set for the children. They now have a solid background for the practice of excessive food intake in their adult years. Then, as a substitute for loneliness, for fatigue, for boredom, for an inner feeling of emptiness, they find temporary surcease by filling up with food. And many fears are born of loneliness, fatigue, boredom, emptiness; the attempt to assuage fear by food intake is well known.

Another important insight is that the same stimuli that trigger people to gain weight may also cause a drastic and pathological loss of weight. Obesity is only one end of a spectrum. The other end is a condition called *anorexia nervosa*, which literally means lack of appetite due to nervous reasons. As with many other medical terms (hypersplenism, intermittent claudication, etc.), it does not give an explanation but is merely descriptive. In anorexia nervosa, which is usually found in adolescent girls, though it does also occur in other women, there is no desire to eat. Food intake is minimal, and body weight can drop drastically. Much as obesity, it is a disturbance of food intake. Thus obesity and anorexia nervosa are both horns of a dilemma—the Scylla and Charybdis of eating—and both have a psychological origin. In fact, it is not extraordinary, though not frequent, for people to go from one extreme to the other, if they survive it. Dietary and psychological ministrations treat both horns of the dilemma, obesity and anorexia nervosa: in obesity, dietary restriction; in anorexia nervosa, dietary plenty.

Extremely rapid reduction of body weight, which unfortunately is what the fat person wants, can precipitate a psychosis if not anorexia nervosa. Thus the *rate* of weight reduction is important in treating both obesity and anorexia nervosa.

One of the important concomitants to obesity is the feeling of being filled—satiety. An obese person has a hunger which he always attempts to sate. But two elements disturb this simple attempt: first, the hunger is not necessarily for food, though he attempts to sate it with food, and second, he is almost never sated. In fact the fat person may actually rarely be either hungry or full. He eats despite the fact that the hunger does not originate in the stomach but in the psyche. The thin person is easily sated, and perhaps therefore remains at a more-or-less constant weight.

While the body is growing, as during childhood and adolescence, there is a clear need to take in more food than is expended for energy. The rest is used for body growth—construction. After full growth is attained, the body is physiologically in a constant state; it does not need to grow. Thus, except for minor adjustments due to ongoing physiological processes, the body weight is and should remain constant. When the food intake is larger than necessary, the rest is stored. But the unfortunate point is that the excess is stored in the form of fat. The body has an almost unlimited capacity to store fat, contrary to its ability to store proteins and carbohydrates. The grand idea of caloric restriction is based on the fact that the stored fat can be used to produce energy needed for daily endeavors during the period that the food intake is smaller than the daily energy needed. It is fortunate that fat can be mobilized to take the place of food, and thus body fat can be lost. This is precisely what is necessary to reduce body weight.

But here is a caution: many people, especially women, would rather talk about reducing weight than actually reducing it. Weight reduction is a fashionable subject to discuss. Often, especially among people who are shy in starting a conversation with strangers, talk about fat reduction breaks the ice. *But it does not take off fat!* And with some, whose inner resources may be rather flat, or whose external interests are rather shallow, it remains one of the few subjects on which they can hold forth in confidence. This is also a factor in self-protection and an attempt to ward off anxiety: the talker-but-not-the-doer should not be blamed.

People usually welcome reasons other than overeating to account for their obesity. It is less than sociably acceptable to admit to overeating, but there is no social unacceptability to being fat due to "glands." As a matter of fact, there are only a few rather far-reaching metabolic causes of obesity, though they are rare. One of them is Cushing's syndrome, a disturbance of the adrenal-pituitary axis. Another is castration, male or female. A third is removal of the frontal lobes of the brain, prefrontal lobotomy. And weight gain frequently follows menopause. But even in the normal events of menopause, weight does not need to be gained if the caloric intake is reduced—often easier said than done.

Obesity has also been produced in rats by obliteration of a certain part of the brain (hypothalamus), after which they eat continuously. Most interestingly, obliteration of another part gives rise to such a lack of appetite that the rats actually starve in the midst of readily available food. This may or may not apply to humans. These centers in the brain are referred to as the appetite or hunger centers. But for all practical purposes, obesity in man is due to excessive food intake, not to destruction of part of the brain, though the reason for the superfluous food intake lies somewhere in the psyche.

How to reduce? To ask an obese person to use will power is naive. The matter is deeper. To ask him to stop eating is absurd. It does not touch the reason for overeating. To shame him into reducing is cruel; it is pointless and merely adds insult to injury.

To give him a diet without psychological support is usually ineffective. To give him motivation is excellent, provided that his psychological constellation accepts it and that a substitute for the urge to overeat is also given. To tell him to go to a psychiatrist may justifiably produce a counterresponse to tell you to go to hell.

But there is hope. You can reduce, and what is even more important, you can retain the new weight or the reduced status. Several instruments are necessary. One is a full-length mirror. Another is clothes—a dress or a suit *which has become too small*. But above all, the most important is your own conviction that loss of weight is imperative.

A scale is not necessary; in fact it may be a detriment. The reason that a scale is a liability is that if the loss of weight, as seen on a scale, is not quick or dramatic, people may become discouraged and relapse. They *see* no positive reinforcement, though it is there. Like drug addicts they relapse when the world does not embrace them for a small accomplishment. Yet even a small accomplishment is a sizable asset because it is a harbinger of the future.

The use of a full-length mirror in the nude, for which there is no substitute, accomplishes several ends. It allows you to take stock not only of your nude appearance but also of the distortions of your posture brought on by the excess weight. The distortion of form can become grotesque even with as little as 20 pounds overweight. But in assessing your appearance before a full-length mirror, do not draw in your abdomen or pose, as for a photograph. The worst delusion is self-delusion.

Also, a mirror, but only a full-length mirror, allows you to see progress in a more telling way than a scale does. A scale offers merely numbers, elements that have to be translated by the imagination. A full-length mirror can show you how both posture and form are improving—and how appearance is enhanced. That is positive reinforcement and will keep motivation on a workable level.

A suit or a dress that was at one time comfortable and now too small is a considerable help. While it cannot be worn every day, it should be put on every week, for comfortably fitting into clothes that were too small for you offers a much more satisfactory reward for reducing, as well as a stimulant to continue, than a scale.

For motivation there is no substitute. If you really want to reduce, rather than just talk about reducing, you have to be sold on the enduring advantage that results from eating less. For example, while it is known that fat people have a shorter life expectancy, you may not be impressed by that; it is too ephemeral to worry about events 20, 30, or 40 years hence.

But you may prize the advantages that an attractive weight will give you while you are in your prime of life. You may find it worthwhile to curtail food intake in exchange for gaining self-confidence (fat people are inevitably self-conscious), or for a better body-image of yourself, or for social acceptability, or even for the banal ability of climbing a flight of steps without the breathlessness that is associated with old age. Or you may want to break the patterns by which you have been enslaved in other areas. If you are fat, that is a splendid way to start.

In any event, the motivation must come from within. We shall not go into the various aspects of physiological health or mental health that weight reduction brings. You may have known them, even vaguely. But if you were not moved by these reasons in the past, no matter how compelling they are, it was due to the fact that you may have had little motivation to reduce body weight.

Should you develop motivation within, you should also be aware of the obstacles that may be in your way; awareness is the first part of victory. For example, if you work at home, or you are a housewife, the temptation to eat is greater, no matter how busy you are. You may find that a change, such as part-time work outside of the house, makes the first few weeks or months easier to implement or to effect your motivation. At times other events in the familial structure conspire against you and you put on weight. For example, children going to college out-of-town or the death of a spouse may be instrumental in gaining weight. Adjustment, by occupation outside of the house, may be the answer to assuaging the frustration or the hollowness produced by such changes.

What may be on the surface an imperceptible change can lead to weight increase. Awareness is necessary here. For example, a reduction of activity such as by the installation of a labor-saving device may lead to an increase in weight. Another example: it was found that typists in the pool of a large corporation gained weight in a four-month period after their manual typewriters were changed to electric ones.

Awareness must also be used in the attempt to add exercise to the sedentary person's weight-reducing regimen. For example, there is a *net gain* in weight if two cocktails are taken after an 18-hole game of golf, which uses about 140 calories of energy expenditure. Two cocktails are equivalent to about 175 calories—a net caloric gain.

Do not ignore the small amount of daily calories that are waiting for you in snacks ready to pounce on you. Always multiply the caloric value by 365, the number of days in the year. For example, only 100 calories a day of some goody amount to 36,500 calories a year—about 9 pounds of fat!

In this connection note the reverse too. While walking is not a dramatic way of reducing—you need to walk 35 miles to reduce one pound of *fat*—it totals up in the course of a year. Daily exer-

Desirable Weights
Weight in Pounds According to Frame
(In Indoor Clothing)

MEN OF AGES 25 AND OVER

Height (with shoes on) 1-inch heels		Small Frame	Medium Frame	Large Frame
Feet	Inches			
5	2	112–120	118–129	126–141
5	3	115–123	121–133	129–144
5	4	118–126	124–136	132–148
5	5	121–129	127–139	135–152
5	6	124–133	130–143	138–156
5	7	128–137	134–147	142–161
5	8	132–141	138–152	147–166
5	9	136–145	142–156	151–170
5	10	140–150	146–160	155–174
5	11	144–154	150–165	159–179
6	0	148–158	154–170	164–184
6	1	152–162	158–175	168–189
6	2	156–167	162–180	173–194
6	3	160–171	167–185	178–199
6	4	164–175	172–190	182–204

cise does reduce weight over the long term, aside from its other benefits.

I shall not set forth a dietary scheme. Lists and books on caloric values and other food values are readily obtainable.

But I want to point out some common practices and to evaluate them. If food is a sedative, and that sedative value will be lost due to caloric restriction, people often take alcohol to "settle down," to unwind. The fallacy here lies in the fact that alcohol contains 7 calories per gram, while proteins and carbohydrates

WOMEN OF AGES 25 AND OVER

Height (with shoes on) 2-inch heels		Small Frame	Medium Frame	Large Frame
Feet	Inches			
4	10	92– 98	96–107	104–119
4	11	94–101	98–110	106–122
5	0	96–104	101–113	109–125
5	1	99–107	104–116	112–128
5	2	102–110	107–119	115–131
5	3	105–113	110–122	118–134
5	4	108–116	113–126	121–138
5	5	111–119	116–130	125–142
5	6	114–123	120–135	129–146
5	7	118–127	124–139	133–150
5	8	122–131	128–143	137–154
5	9	126–135	132–147	141–158
5	10	130–140	136–151	145–163
5	11	134–144	140–155	149–168
6	0	138–148	144–159	153–173

For girls between 18 and 25, subtract 1 pound for each year under 25.
Courtesy of Metropolitan Life Insurance Co.

contain only 4 calories per gram. Alcohol is exceeded in caloric value only by fat, which is equivalent to 9 calories per gram. Moreover, alcohol is both a nervous system depressant and an appetite stimulant. Alcohol gives you empty calories. As a substitute, chew on a carrot or on celery, dipped in a dry wine, *not* a sweet wine with its higher (20 percent) alcoholic content. Dry wines contain less sugar and have an alcoholic content of 10 to 12 percent. Remember, too, that alcohol has no satiety value.

In choosing a diet remember that you want to reduce predominantly fat, not muscle. Hence, be sure to have a diet that is high in protein. One gram of protein per day is required per 2.2 pounds (1 kg) of desired body weight. The high-protein diets with very low carbohydrates are effective, at least for a limited time, until a dietary adjustment has taken place.

People eat more during cold weather or after exposure to cold. The reason is that the heat loss, hence energy loss, is greater and an attempt to make it up may lead to excessive food consumption. If you are cold, and you need to warm up from inside out, a clear, nonfat broth or hot coffee or tea (not hot chocolate) will serve the purpose much more efficiently than food.

In devising your reducing diet you must take into consideration certain factors such as the satiety value of foods (to reduce the feeling of emptiness) in addition to their nutritional value. Fats and proteins sate more easily, hence have a high satiety value; carbohydrates have a smaller satiety value, and alcohol has none! Therefore, some fats with proteins are advisable.

Foods that have a high bulk or residue value are found by some to satisfy the empty feeling. For example, assuming that the caloric values of white bread and whole wheat bread are the same (there is only a small difference), white bread has much less residue than whole wheat bread. So make whatever little bread you eat whole wheat bread.

There is virtually no restriction on the kind of meat as a protein source. But in the attempt to enhance protein intake do not go overboard on eggs, as they are high in cholesterol. You will find that canned raw sauerkraut is an ideal low-calorie roughage producer—a grand pacifier for the empty feeling. It contains only 22 calories per 100 grams (about 3½ oz). If you prefer it boiled, that is fine; but do not make the error of preparing an old-fashioned cooked sauerkraut dish which contains potatoes, peas or lentils, bacon and meat scraps.

Cabbage has about the same caloric and roughage value as

sauerkraut. But it has a mild irritating quality and may increase appetite. As snacks or as a dish you will find the following to be low in calories and quite filling: cooked turnips 27, raw spinach 20, raw mushrooms 16, canned mushrooms 11. (The foregoing figures refer to the number of calories per 100 grams, equivalent to about 3½ oz; which is a generous portion.) But be aware, as the following "innocent" vegetables pack a caloric wallop: dry peas 344, dry lentils 340, lima beans 335—all calories per 100 grams.

Salads are a treat and also a hidden danger. They add needed roughage to the calorie-restricted diet but can undo the good work by a glob of salad dressing. We agree that vinegar alone makes the salad unappetizing. Lemon is better. A teaspoonful of yogurt may be a good substitute for salad dressing—if you like it. You will find, however, that a liberal sprinkling of such spices as tarragon, dill, basil, rosemary, sage, nutmeg, curry, sesame, anise, fennel or caraway seeds, mustard, chili make a salad appetizing. Or you may even douse a salad with vinegar in which one or two of these spices were soaked for some days. You may find these spices to be a new taste sensation which can be used without guilt. (The only exception is chili or mustard, which should be used sparingly, as they are irritating and can increase appetite.)

Ordinarily, salt does not have to be omitted, but it is a good idea to reduce it. Salt binds water in the tissues. Catsup, pickles, Worcestershire and similar sauces are high in salt.

Another form of caloric restriction is the *omnidiet* (*omni* = all). By this device, while eating your normal diet, you observe only two restrictions: (1) you consume only half the quantity you normally eat, and (2) you eliminate *all* alcohol and you further cut down to a very minimum any potatoes and bread from the half-portions you are now eating. This is an effective form of dietary control, and perhaps a less trying one, because the change is not as drastic, and includes most of the familiar foods you normally consume.

The slow reduction of weight is a more satisfying one because there is less discomfort and a greater likelihood of continuing it. Hence, relapses are perhaps less likely. More particularly, slow reduction of body weight will allow your skin to adjust to the new shape; there will be less hanging folds of skin.

A form of do-it-yourself dietary control that is eminently effective is the aversion method. This is probably based upon Oscar Wilde's quip that "To think a thing is to cause it to be," or perhaps more likely William James's epigrammatic "Believe, and your belief will help create the fact."

The aversion method merely requires the user to look upon food with disgust. It is really not hard to do in some high-priced restaurants. Using this approach, a person will eat part of the dish set before him, but will leave the rest. This may well be a more sound method, because obesity is basically caused by a psychically triggered urge to acquire food. Hence, a psychically conditioned sense of disgust should counterbalance the acquisitive urge.

Since in any regimen for reducing body weight dietary intake is reduced, a high-potency multivitamin tablet should be taken daily to prevent a vitamin or micronutrient or trace mineral deficiency.

You have heard of starvation diets. They are enticing regimens for almost instant weight reduction. Under certain conditions they may be desirable, but they must be undertaken only in a hospital under the direct supervision of a physician. And they have substantial drawbacks or dangers.

One drawback is that such rapid loss of weight does not allow the elasticity of the skin to adjust to the new contour. The result: skin hangs on the body in an unsightly way. Another drawback is that muscle as well as fat is lost, which can be a metabolically serious development. Other undesirable effects are acidosis or ketosis and loss of valuable electrolytes.

Another drawback, a more serious one, is the possibility that a psychosis may be precipitated. In fact, psychosis is an ever present danger in a starvation diet. This is not surprising, in view of the fact that obesity is broadly considered the result of neurotic behavior. That is the reason that psychological support and unmistakable self-motivation are as important as dietary restriction for enduring effects.

Perhaps the most effective form of obesity treatment is group therapy, provided that the individual (1) is highly motivated, (2) has found an acceptable group, and (3) is in the care of an acceptable therapist.

Obesity is a national problem of malnutrition. It exceeds any other aspect of malnutrition in the number of individuals affected in the United States. Obesity as well as starvation are dysfunctions of nutrition.

There are few contraindications to reducing obesity due to fat. One is tuberculosis, because it is believed—though by no means certain—that reduction of body weight may reactivate a latent and quiescent case of tuberculosis infection. Perhaps this point is moot because few seriously ill tuberculous individuals are overweight. People who are obese, and have a serious disease—as tuberculosis, heart disease, etc.—should not reduce without the clear advice of their physician.

There are no other conditions in which excessive weight should not be reduced.

Drugs

No drug products, either those available on prescription or over-the-counter without prescription, reduce weight. At best they reduce the desire to eat, and only restriction of dietary intake reduces body weight. None of the products sold as an aid to weight reduction are useful without dietary restriction and without motivation. They may, however, make it easier for a highly motivated person.

Reducing products, as they are commonly called, must be taken with caution, not because they are dangerous—though some can be—but because reliance on them may prevent an individual from seeking more competent methods of weight reduction.

Some of the products available over-the-counter without prescription, as Metrecal, are actually foods. Their advantage in a weight-reduction regimen lies in the fact that by taking them you can precisely measure your caloric intake provided that you conform to directions given. Such products supply proteins, carbohydrates and fats, to assure adequate nutrition, with vitamins and minerals to supplement those that are missing from a restricted diet. In many cases, the total daily food intake consists of these preparations. Variants of these preparations are in cookie form.

The disadvantage of these products lies in the fact that though they are palatable, the sensory component of food intake is missing. Thus early relapse to the regular and unsatisfactory diet is more likely. Some people, however, completely misunderstand the premise on which these preparations are used, and take twice or three times the amounts recommended. The net result is they *gain* weight instead of losing it.

Another type of weight-reducing product consists of wafers with a diet pamphlet. These wafers are high in protein and low in fat, and together with the dietary information and dietary restriction they may be helpful to a strongly motivated person—if it works for him.

An additional form of over-the-counter weight-reducing product consists of candy that contains vitamins and some minerals, notably iron. The principle inherent in this type of product is that candy satisfies, helps sate the user on a reducing diet (about three pieces a day are recommended), and prevents the urge to take more caloric foods. Each piece of candy is high in carbohydrates, moderate in fat and low in protein, and contains 26 calories. If it is found that one, and only one, piece of candy prevents taking more caloric foods—then well and good. But motivation is what gives the successful dieter power to conform to a reducing diet.

Then there is the product in the form of chewing gum or a tablet, which, containing a local anesthetic, benzocaine, is said to reduce the sensory desire for food or to cut down the quantity of its intake. The objective is to substitute one sensation with another, the latter one not leading to caloric intake. These tablets are highly flavored, and as with slimming candy, if this method prevents you from yearning for more food or dessert, well and good. But motivation still is the real answer.

A further method offered by a group of over-the-counter preparations available without prescription is a combination in tablet form of phenylpropanolamine hydrochloride, with vitamins, at times with caffeine, and occasionally with methyl cellulose. None of these, of course, will work without dietary restriction. The vitamins are to substitute for those that are lost because of dietary restriction. The caffeine is a stimulant, which is needed because curtailment of food intake tends to depress. But there is too little caffeine (25 mg) present for that purpose. Methyl cellulose swells in the intestine to give a feeling of bulk to assuage the empty feeling. The trouble is that the place you need it more is in the stomach.

The more important ingredient in these preparations is phenylpropanolamine hydrochloride. Similar to ephedrine, phenylpropanolamine finds its most widespread and dependable uses as an ingredient in nasal or sinus congestion. But one of its actions, though a mild one, is depression of appetite, for which reason it is used in these preparations. The effect is probably too mild in the 25 mg doses administered, but in larger doses it could produce palpitations or wakefulness, and then it would not be available over-the-counter without prescription. Its inclusion in these products is logical, but the degree of the functional effect in reducing appetite may vary from individual to individual. Surely, without caloric restriction it would be useless. No drug is known that takes off fat without causing substantial metabolic upheavals.

An additional method of weight reduction does lessen body weight but not fat; it is a diuretic causing water loss by increasing the flow of urine. *A diuretic does not reduce fat.* Do not consider these products. If you have an accumulation of water in the tissues (edema) see your doctor; it may be due to a dysfunctioning heart.

I should also mention thyroid preparations, which are reputed to be weight reducing. If the thyroid is normal, thyroid tablets will reduce weight only in doses that will be toxic, and which can damage the heart. As a matter of fact, one is worse off after having taken thyroid tablets, whether they reduce or not, because thyroid tablets suppress the natural function of the thyroid gland in the body. The thyroid gland recovers its function—with time. In the event of an underfunction of the thyroid (hypothyroidism) other problems, perhaps more than weight gain, will be present. They should be treated by a physician.

A group of products that create bulk in the intestine—for which reason they are used in constipation—are the hydrophilic colloids, or bulk-producing agents. Creating bulk in the intestine may be helpful when it gives an intestinal sense of fullness. But the sense of fullness is more necessary in the stomach where hunger contractions take place. For some people, however, but with dietary measures, they may be helpful.

As a sweetener saccharin is almost universally used. Cyclamates are no longer available, by government fiat. But some people complain that saccharin leaves a bad aftertaste, yet they do not like unsweetened beverages. The aftertaste can be easily remedied by using only half of that amount of saccharin that was found to be unpleasant. In a short time, perhaps in a week or two, you will become accustomed to and satisfied with partially sweetened beverages. Then it is much easier to drop the use of sweeteners.

The optimum help will be obtained by your own conviction of the need to reduce. To that end you should find helpful one or another of the methods outlined in this chapter. Remember: your objective is to reduce fat, not muscle, and above all to keep down to your reduced weight.

20

WHAT DO CHILDREN NEED IN VITAMINS AND MICRONUTRIENTS?

WHAT CHILDREN NEED in nutrients is simply food. They are continuously expanding and need food both for maintenance of energy and, especially, for growth. Most children are active and, unless they are overweight need a considerable dietary intake. The appetites of boys are notorious.

Do children need vitamins? And if so, how much? The need for the kind of vitamins in children and adults is about the same. Though some authorities hold that neither adults nor children ordinarily need supplemental vitamins and micronutrients, even they prescribe vitamins normally and routinely for infants. Where, then, is the cutoff point? The same reasons given throughout this book as to why adults would do well to take supplemental vitamins and micronutrients apply with equal force to children. But you need not buy chewable vitamins for children unless they object to taking ordinary multivitamin tablets or capsules. When buying vitamins (see table on inside front cover for RDA for children), do get multivitamin-mineral combinations, since iron, zinc and other minerals are particularly necessary for children. See elsewhere in this book for the roles minerals play.

One caution should be noted. Mothers who, for whatever reason, do not bother to plan nutritious meals and allow their children to choose and get their own meals (generally hot dogs and cola drinks) may feel they have discharged their nutritional responsibility by loading the children with vitamins. But vitamins are a supplement; they are not a substitute for food.

Mothers want their children to be healthy and strong. Alertness and growth are largely a function of good nutrition, which may indeed be supplemented by vitamins but is, above all, based on proper food. This is particularly necessary for young people, who have much growing to do. This is one of the reasons that the faddish dieting to which girls frequently resort—often going two or three days without food—is a grave error. Boys too, in trying to lose fat or perhaps in trying to build up to make a football team or similar sports activity, at times practice distorted diets which their weight does not really demand.

Admittedly, it is not easy to get children and teen-agers to eat nutritionally well-designed meals even if a knowledgeable mother painstakingly prepares them. Sweets, desserts, peer pressure and conformity, desire to manipulate parents, psychological reasons, and virtual repugnance to certain foods because mothers repeatedly try to convince them that they are *good-for-you*, are all part of the problem of why children will not eat. Whatever argument you use, never tell a child that *it's-good-for-you*, for that argument will surely fail.

Then if vitamins and micronutrients are not to be used *instead* of thoughtfully prepared meals, how do you get children to eat? The answer is not easy. But a good part of the answer lies in three words: *imagination, magic, fun*. If you use imagination to give food a magical quality and make it fun to eat, the major part of the problem may be solved. But if a food set before youngsters is accompanied by the explanation *it's-good-for-you*, the magic will fall flat, the fun will be gone and your imagination will not have served you well.

Here are a number of suggestions to simplify feeding children with *what's-good-for-them* without letting them know it:

1. *Surprise:*   If you surprise them you may get them to think of you as a friend—which carries a greater cachet than parent. For example, start off an occasional meal with a dessert. Shortly after, they will ask you, "Is that all for dinner?" Then, having asked for more, they will not merely sit as unwilling recipients of what Mother wants them to eat.

2. *Change:*   When you feel you have achieved a workable ritual and all goes well, it is time to change. Find another satisfactory ritual or method. Nothing cloys the palate as much as monotony.

3. *Desserts First:*   There are usually few or no protests about desserts. However, gild the lily, since that may well make the youngster more tractable. For example, if you offer ice cream for dessert, occasionally stick in a lollipop for young children or a licorice stick for older ones. This sort of thing can well reap a bonus when you next set before them a less than favored food.

4. *Banal & Blah:*   Some foods are just pedestrian by nature, and if not liked are hard to disguise. Mix these with a psychological adjunct rather than with another food, where they would probably be recognized. For example, rice, if disliked, can hardly be disguised successfully. Therefore, do not try to hide it but color it pink with an acceptable food coloring and, for a cold drink to accompany the meal, serve pink lemonade. That has the festivity of a circus for the very young.

5. *Put On a Mask:*   Hot, enriched cereals serve a good purpose in winter breakfasts. You can ennoble them just before serving by cutting in small segments of cold fruit, such as pineapple, orange, etc. The surprise may wake up the kids and hurry them

on to school. Or you may be able to convert objections to curiosity
—usually a successful ploy—by cutting in asparagus tips because
these are least expected in a hot cereal. Similarly, an asparagus
spear can be put through a hole cut out in the center of a slice
of Canadian bacon. Another ploy is to cut pieces of toast, dusted
with cinnamon, into circles, squares, or strips to make them look
like cookies. Vegetables can be cut into very small pieces and
mixed into balls of cottage or pot cheese so that they cannot be
picked out. A child may indeed refuse the whole dish, but sometimes he may eat it out of curiosity. At other times, color balls of
cottage or pot cheese: green with spinach juice, brown with
chocolate or cocoa, or pink with beet juice. Still another ploy:
put small wedges of cheddar cheese into segments of orange or
pineapple, or segments of orange or pineapple into cheddar
cheese. It works both ways.

6. *Magic:* Occasionally add a knife-pointful of baking soda
to a glass of tomato juice or to an acid juice such as orange. The
drink then will bubble mildly and offer a bit of magic.

7. *Lip-Smacking:* Children can live on snacks, but they can't
thrive on them. Enrich their snacks with protein, such as peanut
butter, or peanuts in another form. Peanuts are a good, though
not a complete, protein, and are also rich in fat. A tomato that
has been partially scooped out and filled with such goodies as
coarsely ground nuts and small pieces of chocolate make a nutritious snack. As for milk with chocolate syrups added, nothing
is wrong with it as a snack unless it adds more sugar to the diet
than may be wise.

8. *Protein the Hero:* An adequate food intake means a variety
of foods composed of carbohydrates, fats and protein. They
metabolize interdependently. While there is no food that is all-
important to the exclusion of others, children take more easily
to carbohydrates (bread, other starches) and fats (butter) than

to protein. But an adequate protein intake *must* be assured. If there is a protest when you offer undisguised chicken or meat, you may find that the protest will weaken if you serve them in what is ostensibly another dish. For example, mix diced chicken— or soy beans (a complete vegetable protein)—into apple sauce or apple-pineapple-cranberry sauce and serve it as a dessert. It will function nutritionally as well as if served as a main dish.

After you have mastered these artifices you have a chance to feed your children food that is *good-for-them*. You may possibly feel drained from devising such inventions for use in dietary manipulation, but you pay a price for doing your best for your children. That's something your mother has been telling you since *you* were a child.

Finally, remember that children's dietary needs are not the whole story. An emotional input is required as well. Children wilt if deprived of loving parental affection and other attention. But above all they need adequate nutritional input for proper mental as well as physical growth.

READING LIST

Anderson, T. W., D. B. W. Reid and G. H. Beaton, "Vitamin C and the Common Cold: A Double-Blind Trial," *Canad. Med. Assn. J.*, Vol. 107 (1972), p. 503.

Azaroff, D. L., G. L. Curran and W. P. Williamson, "Cholesterol Inhibition by Vanadium in Tumors," *J. Nat. Cancer Inst.*, Vol. 21 (1959), p. 1109.

Bernstein, D. S., N. Sadowsky, M. Hegstead, C. D. Guri, and F. J. Stars, "Osteoporosis in High and Low Fluoride Areas in North Dakota," *J. Amer. Med. Assn.*, Vol. 198 (1966), p. 499.

Bernstein, D. S., N. Sadowsky, M. Hegstead, C. D. Guri, and F. J. Stars, *J. Clin. Endocr.*, Vol. 27 (1967), p. 197.

Buja, L. M. and W. C. Roberts, "Iron Storage Disease," *Am. J. Med.*, Vol. 51 (1971), p. 209.

Cadell, J. L., "Sudden Infant Deaths," *Lancet*, Vol. 2 (1972), p. 258.

Callendar, S. T., "Iron Absorption from Food," *Geront. Clin.*, Vol. 13 (1971), p. 44.

Calhoun, N. A., J. C. Smith, Jr., and K. L. Becker, "Zinc in Bone Formation in Rats." Presented at meetings of the Federation of American Societies for Experimental Biology and Medicine, April 1973.

Chen, L. H., S. Liao and L. V. Packet, "Interaction of Dietary Vitamin E and Protein Level or Lipid Source with Cholesterol in the Rat," *J. Nutr.*, Vol. 102 (1972), p. 729.

Cochrane, W. A., "Excessive Administration of Vitamins," *Canad. Med. Assn. J.*, Vol. 93 (1965), p. 893.

Cohlan, S. Q., "Excessive Intake of Vitamin A as a Cause of Congenital Abnormalities in Rats," *Science*, Vol. 117 (1953), p. 535.

Curran, G. L., D. L. Azaroff and R. E. Bollinger, "Trace Vanadium and Cholesterol Inhibition in Normocholesterolemic Men," *J. Clin. Invest.*, Vol. 38 (1959), p. 1251.

D'Alonzo, C. A. and S. Pell, "Serum Nickel in Infarction," *Arch. Env. Health*, Vol. 6 (1963), p. 381.

Dayton, D. H., "Early Malnutrition and Human Development," *Children* (Nov.–Dec. 1969).

Desforges, J., "Anemia Complicating Pregnancy," *J. Reprod. Med.*, Vol. 10 (1973), p. 111.

Di Cyan, E., *Vitamin E and Aging*. New York: Pyramid Publications, 1972.

Erway, L., L. S. Hurley and A. Fraser, "Neurologic Defect: Manganese in Phenocopy and Prevention of a Genetic Abnormality of Inner Ear," *Science*, Vol. 152 (1966), p. 1766.

Fell, G. S., D. P. Cuthbertson, K. Queen and C. Morrison. Ninth International Congress of Nutrition, Mexico City, 1972.

Flink, E. B., "Magnesium Deficiency Syndrome in Man," *J. Amer. Med. Assn.*, Vol. 160 (1956), p. 1406.

Flink, E. B., R. McCollister, A. S. Prased, J. Melky and R. P. Doe, "Evidence of Clinical Magnesium Deficiency," *Ann. Int. Med.*, Vol. 47 (1957), p. 956.

Goldman, H. I., "Is Dietary Vitamin K Essential?" Ecology of Dysnutrition Seminar, Vitamin Information Bureau, New York, 1972.

Gordonoff, T., "Water-Soluble Vitamins in Excessive Doses," *Schweiz. Med. Wchschr.*, Vol. 90 (1960), p. 726 (as quoted in *J. Amer. Med. Assn.*, Vol. 174 [1960], p. 1672).

Gross, S. and M. V. Guilford, "Vitamin E-Lipid Relationship in Premature Infants," *J. Nutrition*, Vol. 100 (1970), p. 1099.

Hale, F., "Pigs Born Without Eyeballs," *J. Heredity*, Vol. 24 (1933), p. 105.

Hale, F., "Relation of Maternal Vitamin A Deficiency to Microphthalmia in Pigs," *Texas J. Med.*, Vol. 33 (1973), p. 228.

Halstead, J. A. and A. S. Prased, "Zinc Deficiency Syndrome," *Israel Med. J.*, Vol. 22 (1963), p. 307.

Hallbrook, T. and E. Lanner, "Serum Zinc and Healing of Venous Leg Ulcers," *Lancet*, Vol. 2 (1972), p. 780.

Hodges, R. E., *Nutrition Today*. Vol. 5 (1970), p. 11.

Hodges, R. E., "Experimental Vitamin A Deficiency in Man," Western Hemisphere Nutrition Congress III, Miami Beach, 1971.

Holt, L. E., Jr., "Future of Nutrition," *Arch. Dis. Childhood*, Vol. 31 (1956), p. 427 (quoted in *Am. J. Nutrition*, 1958).

Horwitt, M. K., *Vitamins and Hormones*, Vol. 20 (1962), p. 541.

Janes, J. M., J. T. McCall and L. R. Elveback, "Trace Metals in Human Osteogenic Sarcoma," *Mayo Clin. Proc.*, Vol. 47 (1972), p. 476.

Jowsey, J., R. K. Schenck and F. W. Reutter, "Some Effects of Fluoride on Bone Tissue in Osteoporosis," *J. Clin. Endocr.*, Vol. 28 (1968), p. 869.

Laros, R. K., Jr., "Folate Deficiency and Oral Contraceptives," Meeting of Amer. Coll. Obstet. & Gynec., August 1972 (reported in *Family Pract. News*, Sept. 1, 1972).

Leevy, C. M., "Vitamin Therapy," *Drug Therap.*, Vol. 2 (1972), p. 33.

Linthicum, F. H., Jr., "Diagnosis in Cochlear Otosclerosis and Fluoride," *Arch. Otolaryngol.*, Vol. 95 (1972), p. 564.

Lowry, Bessey and Burch, *Proc. Soc. Exp. Biol. Med.*, Vol. 10 (1952), p. 361.

Manocha, S. L., "Malnutrition: Its Impact on Prenatal and Postnatal Life of the Baby," *J. Reprod. Med.*, Vol. 10 (1973), p. 41.

McBean, L. D., J. C. Smith, Jr. and J. A. Halstead, "Zinc and Oral Contraceptives," *Fed. Amer. Soc. Exp. Biol. & Med.*, April 1973.

McCollister, R., E. B. Flink and E. B. Lewis, *Am. J. Clin. Nutr.*, Vol. 12 (1963), p. 415.

Miller, R. F. and R. W. Engel, "Molybdenum," *Fed. Proc.*, Vol. 19 (1960), p. 666.

Monty, K. J., "Effect of Trace Amounts of Molybdenum," Conference Phys. Aspects Water Qual., Washington, D.C., 1960.

Mountain, J. T., F. R. Stockwell, Jr. and H. E. Stockinger, "Inhibitory Effect of Vanadium on Cholesterol Formation in Rabbits," *Proc. Soc. Exp. Biol. Med.*, Vol. 92 (1956), p. 582.

Moynahan, E. J. and P. M. Barnes, "Zinc Deficiency and Synthetic Diet," *Lancet*, Vol. 1 (1973), p. 676.

Naess, K., *J. Norweg. M. Assn.*, Vol. 92 (1972), p. 33.

Nair, P. P., E. Mezev, H. S. Murti, J. Quartner and A. I. Mendeloff, "Vitamin E in Human Porphyrin Metabolism in Man," *Arch. Int. Med.*, Vol. 128 (1971), p. 411.

National Dairy Council, *Dairy Council Digest,* Vol. 5 (1968), p. 26.

Ochsner, A., *New Eng. J. Med.,* Vol. 271 (1964), p. 211.

Pauling, L., *Proc. Nat. Acad. Sci.,* Vol. 67 (1970), p. 1643.

Peer, L. A., H. W. Gordon and W. G. Bernhard, "The Experimental Production of Congenital Deformities and Their Possible Prevention in Humans," St. Barnabas Med. Center, Newark, N.J. Sponsored by John A. Hartford Foundation, New York.

Perla, D. and J. Marmorston, *Natural Resistance and Clinical Medicine.* Boston: Little, Brown & Co., 1941.

Pories, W. J., J. H. Henzel, T. N. Caris, C. G. Rab and W. H. Strain, "Promotion of Healing by Oral Zinc Therapy," *Clin. Med.* Vol. 00 (1967).

Pories, W. J., J. H. Henzel, C. G. Rab and W. H. Strain, "Acceleration of Wound Healing in Man by Zinc Sulfate Given by Mouth," *Lancet,* Vol. 1 (1967), p. 121.

Pories, W. J., J. H. Henzel, C. G. Rab and W. H. Strain, "Acceleration of Wound Healing," *Ann. Surg.,* Vol. 165 (1967), p. 432.

Prasad, A. S., *Zinc Metabolism.* Springfield, Illinois: Charles C Thomas, 1966.

Ritchie, J. H., M. B. Fish, V. McMasters and M. Grossman, "Edema and Hemolytic Anemia in Premature Infant. A Vitamin E Deficiency Syndrome," *New Eng. J. Med.,* Vol. 279 (1968), p. 1185.

Roe, D. A., "Drug Induced Vitamin Deficiencies," *Drug Therap.,* Vol. 3 (1973), p. 23.

Rosenstock, H. A., D. G. Simons and J. S. Meyer, "Chronic Manganism," *J. Amer. Med. Assn.,* Vol. 217 (1971), p. 1354.

Schroeder, H. A., "Trace Metals," *J. Chron. Dis.,* Vol. 18 (1965), p. 217.

Schroeder, H. A., "Losses of Vitamins and Trace Minerals Resulting from Processing and Preservation of Foods," *Am. J. Clin. Nutr.,* Vol. 24 (1971), p. 562.

Schroeder, H. A., "Renal Cadmium and Essential Hypertension," *J. Amer. Med. Assn.,* Vol. 187 (1964), p. 358.

Schroeder, H. A. and J. J. Balassa, "Cadmium," *J. Chron. Dis.,* Vol. 14 (1961), p. 236.

Schroeder, H. A., J. J. Balassa and I. H. Tipton, "Chromium," *J. Chron. Dis.,* Vol. 15 (1962), p. 941.

Schroeder, H. A., J. J. Balassa and I. H. Tipton, "Manganese," *J. Chron. Dis.*, Vol. 19 (1966), p. 545.

Schroeder, H. A., J. J. Balassa and I. H. Tipton, "Nickel," *J. Chron. Dis.*, Vol. 15 (1962), p. 51.

Schroeder, H. A., J. J. Balassa and I. H. Tipton, "Lead," *J. Chron. Dis.*, Vol. 14 (1961), p. 408.

Schroeder, H. A., J. J. Balassa and I. H. Tipton, "Tin," *J. Chron. Dis.*, Vol. 17 (1964), p. 483.

Schroeder, H. A., J. J. Balassa and I. H. Tipton, "Titanium," *J. Chron. Dis.*, Vol. 16 (1963), p. 55.

Schroeder, H. A. and M. Mitchener, "Selenium and Tellurium," *J. Nutr.*, Vol. 101 (1971), p. 1531.

Schroeder, H. A., A. P. Nason, I. H. Tipton and J. J. Balassa, "Zinc," *J. Chron. Dis.*, Vol. 20 (1967), p. 179.

Schwarz, K., *Nutr. Rev.*, Vol. 18 (1960), p. 1963.

Schwarz, K., Ninth International Congress of Nutrition, Mexico City, 1972.

Schwarz, K., "Trace Amounts of Selenium," Conference on Physiologic Aspects of Water Quality, Washington, D.C., 1960.

Schwarz, K. and W. Mertz, "Chromium—The Glucose Tolerance Factor," *Arch. Biochem. and Biophysics*, Vol. 85 (1959), p. 292.

Shittle, C. R., "Sudden Crib Deaths," *Lancet*, Vol. 2 (1971), p. 1280.

Stitt, F. W., M. D. Crawford, D. G. Clayton and J. N. Morris, "Clinical and Biochemical Indicators of Cardiovascular Disease Among Men Living in Hard and Soft Water Areas," *Lancet*, Vol. 1 (1973), p. 122.

Stockinger, H. E., "Trace Amounts of Vanadium," Conference on Physiologic Aspects of Water Quality, Washington, D.C., 1960.

Streiff, R. R., "Folate Deficiency and Oral Contraceptives," *J. Amer. Med. Assn.*, Vol. 214 (1970), p. 40.

Swift, P. G. F. and J. L. Emery, *Lancet*, Vol. 2 (1972), p. 871.

Tappel, A. L., *Geriatrics*, Vol. 23 (1963), p. 97.

Vallee, B. L., "The Metabolic Role of Zinc," *J. Amer. Med. Assn.*, Vol. 162 (1956), p. 1054.

Vallee, B. L., "Zinc Deficiency," *Phys. Rev.*, Vol. 39 (1959), p. 443.

Vallee, B. L., W. E. C. Wacker and D. D. Ulmer, "Magnesium Deficiency Tetany Syndrome in Man," *New Eng. J. Med.*, Vol. 262 (1960), p. 155.

Wacker, W. E. C., "Trace Amounts of Zinc," Conference on Physiologic Aspects of Water Quality, Washington, D.C., 1960.

Williams, H. T. G., D. Fenna and R. A. Macbeth, "Alpha Tocopherol in Intermittent Claudication," *Surg. Gynec. Obstet.*, Vol. 132 (1971), pp. 662–666.

Williams, R. J., *Nutrition Against Disease.* New York: Pitman Publishing Co., 1971.

Wohl, M. G. and R. S. Goodhart, *Modern Nutrition in Health and Disease,* 4th Ed. Philadelphia: Lea and Febiger, 1968.

Yacowitz, H., "Urine Excretion of Minerals in Obese Humans on Normal and High Protein Low-Calorie Diets." Paper delivered at 1973 meeting of American Society of Experimental Biology.

INDEX

Acne, vitamin A and, 46, 50
Adenosine triphosphate (ATP), 110, 130, 163
Adolescence, 35, 46, 183
Adrenal corticosteroids, 123
Adrenal glands
  obesity and, 184
  pantothenic acid and, 71, 73
  vitamin A and, 47
  vitamin C and, 81, 84
Aged
  calcium and, 163
  deficiencies in, 34
  diet of, 33, 34
  water need in, 171–72
Aging
  calcium loss and, 123
  micronutrients and, 113, 118, 122, 127
  vitamin C and, 83
  vitamin D and, 177
  vitamin E and, 96–97
Alcoholism, 26–27, 36
  brain damage in, 129–30
  cholesterol and, 26–27
  cobalt and, 120
  iron and, 125
  magnesium deficit in, 129–30
  micronutrient overload and, 108–9
  obesity and, 188–89
  pantothenic acid deficit in, 71
  pellagra and, 65
  potassium deficit in, 167
  pyridoxine deficit in, 69–70

Alcoholism (*Cont.*)
  riboflavin and, 63
  thiamine deficit and, 58–59
  vitamin C and, 84
  vitamin K and, 101
  zinc loss in, 139–40, 143
Allergy, 86, 177
"American" diet, 33
American Institute of Nutrition, 41
American Medical Association, 41, 75
Amino acids, 23
  carcinoid and, 37–38
  essential, 23
  nicotinic acid cycle and, 37–38
  pellagra and, 65
  pyridoxine and, 70
Aminopterin, 175
Anderson, Terence W., 114
Anemia
  cobalt and, 104
  fish-tapeworm, 79
  folic acid and, 74–76
  intrinsic factor and, 78
  iron and, 109, 125, 126–27
  liver ingestion and, 24
  in pregnancy, 156–57
  vitamin B_{12} and, 77–78
  vitamin E and, 97
Animals
  birth defects in, 154, 158–60
  differences in responses of, 20
  experimental use of, 20
  micronutrient deficit in, 105

Enzymes (*Cont.*)
  definition of, 20, 153
  magnesium and, 110, 130
  manganese and, 132
  metabolic errors and, 68
  micronutrients and, 109–10, 112
  milk and, 29
  molybdenum and, 133
  pantothenic acid and, 72
  porphyria and, 96
  pyridoxine and, 69
  thiamine and, 60, 152
  zinc and, 141–42
Ephedrine, 195
Epilepsy, 76
Epithelium, 45, 46
Ergosterol, 89
Essential, definition of, 23
Ester, 51
Ethionine, 21
Ethnicity, 29–30, 33
Evans, Herbert McLean, 12
Exercise, obesity and, 187–88
Eye(s)
  riboflavin and, 63
  thiamine and, 59
  vitamin A and, 43, 44–45, 49, 107
  vitamin C and, 84
Eyelid inflammation, 68

Fairleigh Dickinson University, 25
Fat
  diets and, 25
  obesity and, 180
  polyunsaturated, 27
  selenium and, 135, 136
  storage of, 183
  thiamine and, 60
  vitamin A and, 43, 44, 48, 51
  vitamin D and, 89

Fat-soluble vitamins. *See also* Vitamins A, D, E, K.
  deficiency of, 44, 48
  malabsorption and, 34
  in milk, 28
Fatty acids, 58, 64
Fell, Gordon S., 142
Fertility, 93
Fish
  calcium and phosphorus in, 164
  iodine in, 125
  liver oil, 51, 89
  micronutrients in, 117, 137
  sodium and potassium in, 170
  thiaminase in, 174
Flink, E. B., 129, 130
Flour milling, 111
Fluoride, 123
Fluorine, 122–24
  dental caries and, 12, 122
  sources of, 28, 124
Folate, 74, 76
Folic acid (folacin), 74–77
  anemia and, 74–76
  antivitamin, 175
  in pregnancy, 157
  sources, 28, 76–77
Folinic acid, 74
Food(s). *See also* Diet(s).
  anxiety and, 180
  biotin in, 74
  cadmium in, 117
  calcium in, 164
  cobalt in, 120
  chromium in, 119
  cooking or processing of, 32, 33, 53, 77, 86, 111
  copper in, 122
  dislikes, 24, 32
  excessive intake of, 35
  fluorine in, 124
  folic acid in, 76–77

Micronutrients (*Cont.*)
toxicity of, 104, 107–9, 145, 177–78
in water, 114
Milk, 27–30
acne and, 46
breast-feeding, 163
butterfat in, 27, 29
calories in, 27, 29
cholesterol in, 27
intolerance, 29–30
micronutrients in, 28
nonfat dry, 29
sodium and sugar in, 29
vitamins in, 28, 54, 62, 66, 91
Milligram, 61, 78
Milling, 111
Mineral oil, 48
Mineral tablets, 107–8
Minerals, 162–70
trace. *See* Micronutrients.
Molybdenum, 133–34, 147
copper and, 121, 133
in milk, 28
Mountain, J. T., 139
Mouth dryness, 43
Mouth lesions, 63, 65
Moynahan, E. J., 141
Mucous membrane, 45, 97
Murray, T. Keith, 41, 42
Muscle, 25, 95
minerals and, 130, 167

Naess, Knut, 97
Nair, P. P., 96
National Academy of Sciences–National Research Council, 38, 39
Nerve vitamins, 56
Nervous system
B vitamins and, 65, 66, 68, 75
calcium and, 163

Nervous system (*Cont.*)
magnesium and, 130
manganese and, 132
phosphorus and, 163
Neuritis, retrobulbar, 59
Newborn
hemorrhagic disease of, 100
jaundice, 177
Niacin (nicotinic acid), 64–67
actions of, 65–66
alcohol and, 36
antivitamins, 175
cycle, 37–38
pellagra and, 64–65
sources of, 28, 62, 66–67
tryptophan conversion to, 65–66
Niacinamide, 65, 66
Nickel, 134–35
Nicotinamide, 65
Nicotinic acid. *See* Niacin.
Niedermeiser, William, 115
Night blindness, 59
Nucleic acids, 113, 160–61
B vitamins and, 69, 75, 78
Nutrition. *See also* Diet(s).
for children, 198–202
in disease, 151
experimental, in animals, 20
inadequate intake, 34
selection of food in, 23–24
water and, 24

Obesity, 179–97
alcohol and, 188–89
aversion method for, 192
benzocaine for, 195
brain function and, 184
bulk producers and, 196
candy for, 194–95
cause of, 180

Thiamine (*Cont.*)
alcohol and, 36, 58–59
antivitamins, 21, 174–75
carbohydrates and, 58, 60
deficiency, 58–60
enzymes and, 60, 152
metabolite conversion of, 21
pyrophosphate, 21
sources of, 28, 61–62
strength of, expression of, 61
stress and, 59–60
surgery and, 60–61
thyroid activity and, 35
ultilization of, 60
Threonine, 23
Throat dryness, 43
Thyroid gland
iodine and, 12, 124
obesity and, 196
vitamin B₁ and, 35
Tin, 138
Titanium, 104
Toxicity, 145
barium, 146
cadmium, 117
cobalt, 119–20
micronutrients, 145, 177–78
vitamin, 49–50, 176–78
Trace metals, minerals, or elements. *See* Micronutrients.
"Traffic signs," 37
Transaminase, serum, 37
Transferin, 127
Transketolase, 37, 60
Trans-retinoic acid, 46
Triglycerides, 27
"Trojan Horse" syndrome, 173–174
Tryptophan, 23, 37–38, 65–66, 70
Tuberculosis, obesity and, 193
Tungsten, 134
Tyrosine, 23

Unavailable, definition of, 111
U.S. Recommended Daily Allowances (U.S. RDA), 38–39
Unutilizable, definition of, 111
Uric acid, 24, 25
Urination, 35, 36

Valine, 23
Vallee, B. L., 129
Vanadium, 113, 138–39, 147
Vegetables
calcium in, 164
micronutrients in, 128, 132, 138
phosphorus in, 164
in reducing, 190–91
sodium and potassium in, 168–170
vitamin A in, 53, 54
vitamins B in, 62, 70, 73, 77, 79
vitamin C in, 87
Vegetarians, cobalt deficit and, 120
Viets, Franck J., Jr., 144
Vision, 43, 44–45, 59, 107
Vitamin(s), 12
birth defects and, 154, 157
for children, 198–202
deficiencies. *See* Deficiencies; *also* specific vitamins.
definition of, 19
dietary, 32–33
drug taking and, 175–76
excretion of excessive, 35
labeling of, 22
in pregnancy, 159–60
as sentinels, 150–51
supplementation of, 30–33, 36
Vitamin A, 40–55
absorption of, 51
acid, 46
acne and, 46, 50
birth defects and, 154

Vitamin E (*Cont.*)
  sources of, 28, 98
  supplementation, 98
Vitamins F and G, 58
Vitamin H, 73
Vitamin K, 99–101
  alcoholics and, 101
  antibiotics and, 36
  antivitamin, 175
  deficiency, 99–100
  discovery of, 12
  function of, 100–101
  sources of, 28, 101
  supplementation, 101
  toxicity, 177
Vitamins M, P, and U, 57
Vitamin Y, 58
Vomiting, salt loss and, 166

Wafers, reducing, 194
Water, 171–72
  diuretics and, 196
  fluorine in, 122, 124
  hard, 139
  micronutrients in, 108, 114
  nutrition and, 24
  soft, 114
  in weight reduction, 25
Watercress, 88
Water-soluble vitamins, 58
  in milk, 28
  in pregnancy, 177
Weight reduction, 183–97. *See also* Obesity.

Weights, desirable, charts of, 188–89
Wernicke's syndrome, 59
Western Hemisphere Nutrition Congress, 41
Wheat germ, 80
Williams, Robert R., 12
Williams, Roger J., 85
Wilson's disease, 121, 122
Wine, 102
Winick, Myron, 155

Xerophthalmia, 45

Yacowitz, Harold, 25
Yeast, B vitamins and, 62, 80

Zinc, 139–44, 147
  alcoholism and, 139–40, 143
  cadmium and, 143
  cancer and, 115
  copper and, 105, 121, 122, 133–34
  deficiency of, 140–41, 143–44
  diets and excretion of, 25
  earth eating and, 140–41
  enzymes and, 141–42
  healing of wounds and, 141–42, 147
  heart and, 143
  salts, 146
  senses of taste and smell and, 142
  sources of, 28, 144